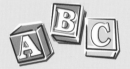

The Toddler Bistro

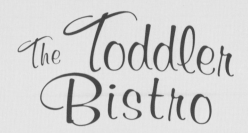

ABC

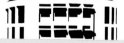

the Toddler Bistro

**Child–Approved Recipes and
Expert Nutrition Advice for the Toddler Years**

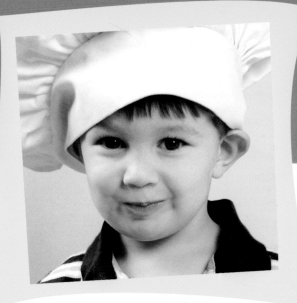

Christina Schmidt, M.S. Nutrition

Bull Publishing Company

Boulder, Colorado

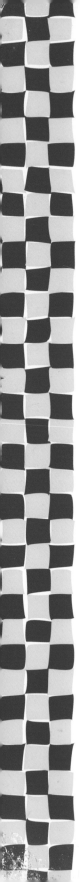

Bull Publishing Company

P.O. Box 1377
Boulder, CO 80306
(800) 676-2855
www.bullpub.com

Book design and production by Shannon Bodie, Lightbourne, Inc.

Design concept by John Betlejewski

Illustrations by Steve Veach

Photography by Peter McQuarry, McQuarry Photography (children and recipes)

Printed in Canada by Friesens

Distributed to the Trade by
Independent Publishers Group
814 North Franklin Street
Chicago, IL 60610

Library of Congress Cataloging-in-Publication Data

Schmidt, Christina, 1970-
 The toddler bistro : child-approved recipes and expert nutrition advice for the toddler
years / Christina E. Schmidt.
      p. cm.
 Includes bibliographical references and index.
 ISBN 978-1-933503-19-6
 1. Toddlers--Nutrition. 2. Cookery (Baby foods) I. Title.

 RJ216.S3985 2009
 613.2083'2--dc22

                              2009030089

Acknowledgments a la Mode

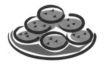

My loving family—Grandma B., mom Susan, sister Gretchen, brother Pete, and husband Neil

My little tasters—Adam, Grant, Evan, Trent, and, of course, my dog Cedar

My forever friends—Neil, Robyn, Karol, Mary, Anne, Erika, Kalai, and Luisa

My genius designer—John Betlejewski, Design Touch

My imaginative illustrator—Steve Veach, Veach Illustration and Design

My gifted and patient photographer—Peter McQuarry, McQuarry Photography

My brilliant reviewers—Iris Castañeda-Van Wyk, M.D., Daniel Brennan, M.D., Myron I. Liebhaber, M.D., Erika Conner, R.D., Patti Stoffers, C.N.P., Robyn Shields, D.D.S.

My publishing dream team—Jim, Betsy, George, Shannon, and Faith

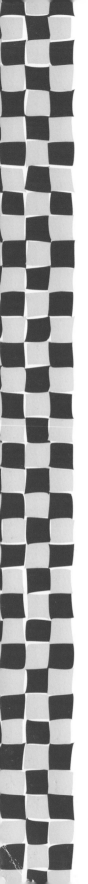

The Menu

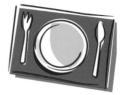

Chef – Christina E. Schmidt, M.S., N.E.

Starters ... *Toddler eating trends and tips for dealing with them* — 1

First Course ... *Food safety* — 17

Second Course ... *Family environmental health* — 41

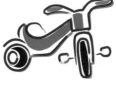

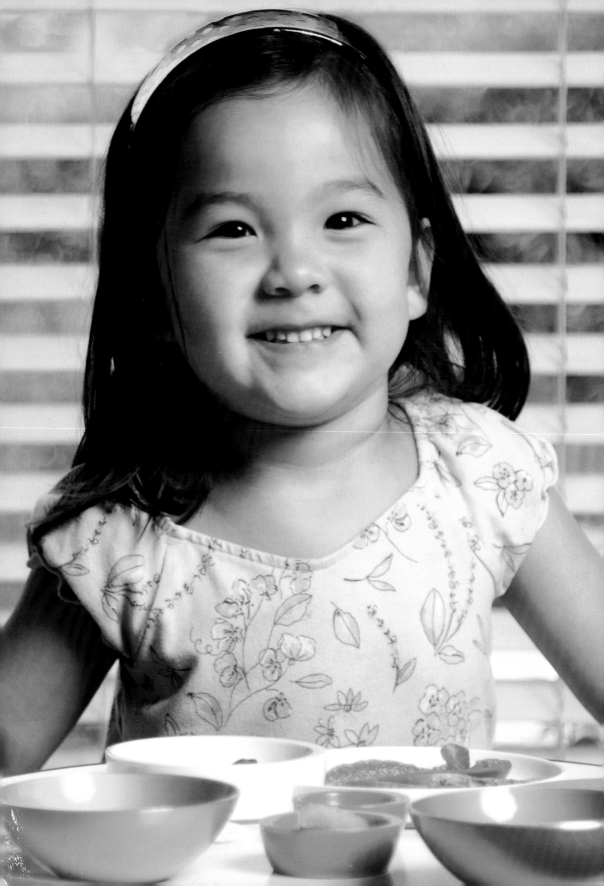

The Birth

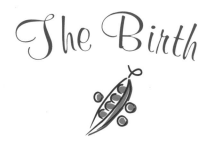

Of the Toddler Bistro

My research and writing about toddler nutrition was not so much inspired by my own intellectual curiosity about nutrition, although I have that in spades. It was literally demanded by the multitudes of confused and bewildered parents out there who wanted to know how and what in the world to feed their toddlers. It seemed as if I couldn't write fast enough!

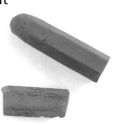

The Birth

If your baby is already into the toddler years, you probably know what I'm talking about. Most parents with toddlers find that at some point mealtimes are a bit challenging, to say the least. You have the best of intentions to serve healthy and nutritious foods but lose steam when all of your hours of food preparation result in your toddler either rejecting or acting completely oblivious to your marvelous meal. You might get stuck in a recipe rut, making or buying the one thing you know your child will eat.

If this eating scenario sounds familiar or happens at some point in the future, never fear and never give up. This, too, shall pass, and it does. As soon as you think that your toddler is disgusted by a certain food, you turn around the next day and find him or her eating it, probably off someone else's plate. Why? Because that's what they do. What should you do? You may laugh in exasperation at this, but please relax and keep the faith. If you keep offering healthy foods, your efforts will pay off in the long run. So, welcome to the Toddler Bistro, where I'll help you with the short run!

The Toddler Bistro menu is your gourmet tour to healthy feeding. At the top of the menu, Starters introduces you to personality developments that may affect your toddler's eating habits and explains how to deal with them. The First and Second Course chapters cover food and environmental safety issues that relate to cooking and eating. Entrées offers a collection of easy-to-prepare and yummy toddler-tested recipes that the whole family will enjoy. These recipes are fresh variations on less-healthy kid favorites, as well as some creative new ideas to help inspire you in the kitchen and at the market. Many of the recipes also include a vegan version.

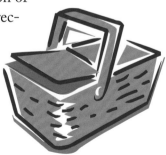

Á la Carte boasts a tantalizing selection of information about important food groups, nutrients, and supplements to enhance your toddler's health. Read all about today's health trends that are important to our future generations and discover tips on how to manage those trends in the Extras chapter. Last but not least is, of course, Desserts, your fun final course. This chapter ensures that you'll graduate from toddler-feeding training with honors. Don't even think about cheating and reading the end first!

All in all, my Toddler Bistro is about empowering you with nutritional knowledge, recipes, and appendices filled with food-brand shopping tips and online resources so that you can confidently launch your toddler onto a healthy, happy path to good eating.

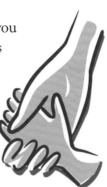

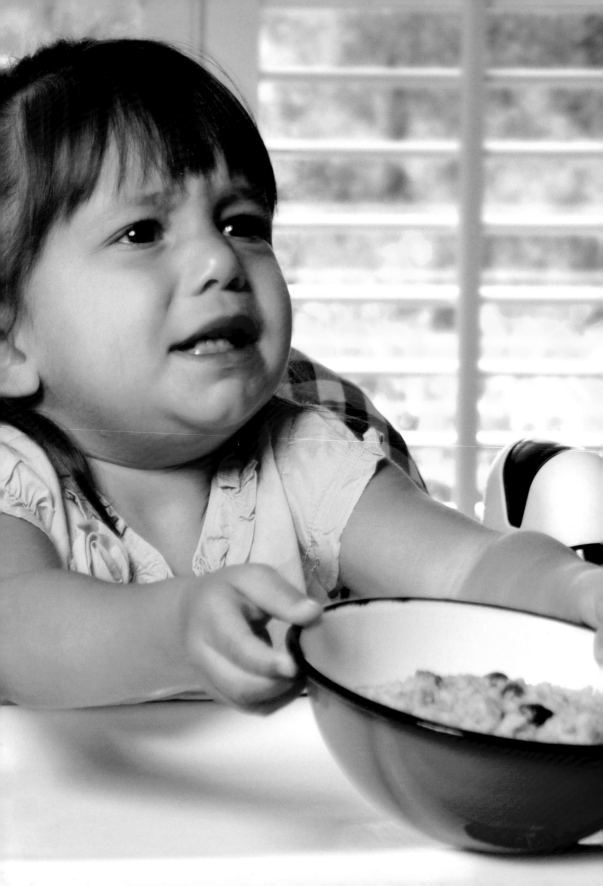

Starters

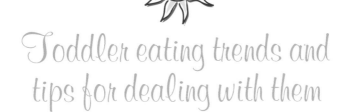

Toddler eating trends and tips for dealing with them

> "I can't get my toddler to drink milk!"

> "My baby used to love eating vegetables and now he won't touch them!"

> "I go to all this work making special meals for my toddler and they just go to waste."

Yes, for some parents of toddlers those honeymoon days, when their sweet babies smile and happily swallow whatever baby food is waved in front of them, are now over. Toddlers will demand any food at the store that is brightly packaged with toys inside, whether or not it's good for them. Some toddlers actually eat their fruits and vegetables enthusiastically while parents of less complaisant eaters stand by in amazement. What's going on? Maybe your challenging toddler is karmic payback for your own stubbornness as a child, but more realistically, your toddler's approach to food follows some general trends after the first birthday.

Personalities

It's a good idea to know a bit about the character and taste of your clientele before opening your Toddler Bistro!

A big new world of discovery surrounds toddlers every day, and they need to feel in control of some part of it. They love things their size: tables, chairs, utensils, plates, and food servings.

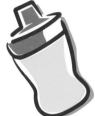

You'll discover some or all of these personality traits evolving in your toddler. They may bewilder you, but these traits signify a positive stage of development that you can still use to your advantage when it comes to introducing healthy foods.

- **Declaring independence!**
  Toddlers like their own space and may eat more of your lovingly prepared meals if they have their own toddler-sized eating area for some meals or snacks.

- **Saying lots of "no's," whether or not they make sense!**
  Turn away from tantrums. Attention only guarantees more. "No" is the name of the game, so offering limited choices of foods and activities can help you outsmart your little rebel. Tantrums are just a toddler's way of testing your limits. You can lose it later, when you're alone, but keep your composure and ignore the tirade. It will pass!

- **Understanding one point of view—theirs!**
  It's terrific that your toddler asserts an opinion, as long as it is within your set of rules. Your toddler's outlook will change if yours stays consistent.

- **Having a short attention span.**

  Focusing on food is sometimes an insurmountable task for toddlers. They may be "grazers" who rarely sit and finish a meal and would rather snack throughout the day. Don't worry: If you make progress with one out of three meals and some snacks, you are doing very well. Keep up a consistent mealtime and snack routine despite your little one's obliviousness to the plate.

- **Being highly unpredictable—expect the unexpected!**

  One day it's "I don't want it," and the next week they can't get enough of it, or vice versa. Whatever it is, as long as you keep offering healthy options to your toddler, it's a win/win situation.

- **Wanting to please their peers.**

  Hopefully your toddler has playmates who love vegetables and detest fried potatoes, never play roughly, and always say thank you. However, if that's not the case, keep in mind that your child's actions among playmates are more about socialization than food—or play styles or manners. Encourage the positive behaviors they display in groups and maintain your stand on the negative ones.

- **Mimicking both parents and peers.**

  Be a role model for healthy eating and manners in front of your toddler. Even if the results are not immediate, being a role model will pay off in the long run!

Bistro Basics

Commit to being copied! Now is the time when you can make the most difference in your toddler's eating behavior. Studies show that food preferences are shaped between the ages of two and three.

Palate preferences

Are there ways to prepare food that are appealing to toddler tastes? Below are some general features of food that most young diners seem to prefer.

- **Food temperature**—Not too hot, not too cold, but just right, which is warm or close to room temperature.
- **Consistency**—Smooth, not lumpy.
- **Texture**—Raw to slightly cooked rather than fully cooked vegetables. Toddler texture preferences will also depend on whether they have enough teeth to chew raw foods.

Absent appetites

In general, your toddler's growth rate slows in comparison to the first year, so don't be alarmed if the insatiable hunger of infancy fades into a more casual interest in food. Appetite busters common to toddlers are grazing, teething, colds, ear infections, fatigue, stress, inactivity, filling up on fluids like milk or juice before a meal, or short attention spans. On the other hand, your toddler may wolf down everything in sight during a growth spurt or when coming off a two-meal food fast. Due to toddlers' fluctuating appetites, skipping a meal or two is normal, but check with your health care provider if the food fast is unusual and excessive.

Toddler Tips

It is very important to allow toddlers to listen to their internal hunger cues. Healthy toddlers self-regulate their food intake surprisingly well!

Bistro Basics
Clarify the "clean the plate" concept.
Your job is to choose the menu and dining times. Your toddler may decide which of your daily specials to eat, if any. Chefs may try requesting "courtesy bites."

Picky palates . . . They like it how they like it!

Assuming that certain foods are the enemy is a normal way for toddlers to initiate their independence and need for control. One theory suggests that pickiness is an instinct that evolved to prevent Stone Age babies from sticking poisonous prehistoric bugs or plants in their mouths.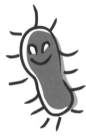

The Chef suggests these strategies to improve your toddler's eating during a "selective eating" stage:

- Avoid stereotyping your toddler as picky and make a mental note to not be a role model for finicky eating in front of your toddler.

- Don't overreact, scold, bribe, beg, or reward with a treat to get your toddler to eat. Overcontrolling your toddler's eating behavior turns down the volume of the natural internal cues for hunger and fullness. Studies show that unpressured children will instinctively balance their diet!

- Prevent your toddler from filling up on excessive fluids before meals. Offering sips of water or milk to quench thirst is fine. Two full sippy cups before a meal, however, may be the reason the plate goes back to the kitchen untouched.

- Allow your little purists their eccentricities, such as not wanting foods to touch each other, but avoid the short-order chef syndrome. Catering to special requests at each meal will reinforce finicky behavior. Offer limited choices (broccoli or carrots?), and serve one sure winner with each meal. Try this trick: Offer a tablespoon of the suspect food with an old reliable favorite when your toddler is hungriest. It works!

- Don't obsess about getting all of the food groups into your toddler daily; think weekly instead. Toddlers' diets magically tend to balance out nutritionally over a few days to a week (see Expanding the Palate, page 7, and Toddler Tasting Tricks, page 9).

- Pack each bite with nutrition, because you never know if it will be the last of that meal or day. Your goal is to maximize the opportunity for your toddler to eat healthy foods!

Food fixations

The love of ritual may provoke your toddler to take the term "comfort food" to the extreme. If your toddler turns type A on you and only certain foods such as white foods are in, it's okay—you can handle it.

Try subtle variations of the original dish your toddler has elected as the best and only edible food of all time. For example, serve other white foods from the Toddler Bistro's White Foods Menu:

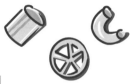

- **Bread**
- **Flour tortillas**
- **Pasta**
- **Potatoes**
- **Milk***
- **Yogurt**
- **Cheese**
- **Cottage cheese**

- **Eggs, hard-boiled***
- **Cauliflower**
- **Parsnips**
- **Jicama**
- **White bean purée**
- **Tofu**

* See First Course, Allergy Alert, page 18, and Beverage Briefs, page 21.

If the food of the moment that your toddler worships is nutritious, let it go! Ride out the fixation for a few weeks, then try the old "Oops, it's all gone and I forgot to buy it" line and substitute a similar dish.

If the phase lasts more than a couple of months, call your health care provider.

Expanding the palate

Learning about new foods is an important part of childhood. Toddlers are naturally curious and want to eat, so here are some ways to extend their dietary horizons.

- Serve new foods casually, "grandfathering" them in with the old. Making a big deal out of a new food may provoke your toddler to instantly reject it. Every few days to few weeks, introduce an unfamiliar food to a meal with an old reliable and let your toddler get used to the look and taste of the new offering.

- Tasting needs the test of time. Most parents only reintroduce a food three to five times, while studies show that it takes eight to fifteen times for new foods to get a green light from toddlers. Don't give up: Keep reintroducing the food every few days.

- Be the role model for tasting *and* liking the food! You truly are the primary influencer of how your toddler relates to and accepts various foods. Your toddler's food preferences directly relate to what you like, as well as to the variety of choices you offer on the menu.

- If you grow it, they will eat it. Toddlers love to eat foods that they have witnessed from seed to plate.

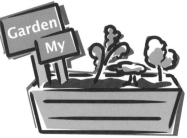

- Take a trip to your local farm. Some farms offer tours for kids to help them connect to their natural environment and learn how food is grown and harvested.

- Go shopping together at farmers' markets or grocery stores. Allow your toddler to see, feel, and touch produce. Use this time to teach about healthy foods. Talk about all of the different kinds of fruits and vegetables—about their flavors, colors, shapes, seasons, and how they grow.

- Cultivate a culinary kid! Think about it: Your skills in the kitchen, or lack thereof, influence your food choices. Toddlers love to help out and to create and therefore might be inclined to eat! You can enlist your toddler, starting at around two years of age, to wash produce, peel bananas, stir and mix, sprinkle spices, help measure and pour ingredients, tell you when the timer goes off, hand you ingredients, decorate and arrange dishes, and help clean up. Try creating a menu together!

- Keep your sous-chef away from the stove and electric appliances. Make sure that your little chef doesn't handle raw meats or raw eggs.

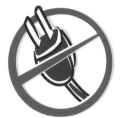

Toddler tasting tricks

It's time to get creative in inspiring your toddler to get excited about eating! Remember those Mickey Mouse pancakes you loved? Here are some more ways to make food fun and enticing.

- Become a food artist. Design and use colorful foods on the plate. Arrange green beans into a pine tree or a spider, or make a fruit or vegetable rainbow.

- Name it something new! Broccoli can be trees, peas can be baseballs, oatmeal raisin cereal can be ant cereal, spaghetti and cheese can be slimy worms, tomato slices can be hot-rod wheels, and colorful fruit slices or chopped veggies can be rainbows. If your toddler loves fries or cookies, try cutting veggies and other less-favored foods into that shape and calling them "veggie fries" or "carrot cookies."

- Shape and sculpt. Use a fun cookie cutter for cheese, sandwiches, or fruit slices. Make teddy bear–shaped pancakes. Swirl mashed sweet potato with yogurt. Buy fun pasta shapes (stars, suns, moons, animals). Make a "mini" version. Silver-dollar-sized pancakes, mini-muffins, and mini-pizzas appeal to those little hands!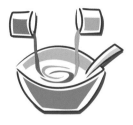

- Offer two to three choices from a certain food group. Let your toddler choose between red pepper strips or carrot sticks. They love to have an option.

- Tell a tale. "Once upon a time, a big bird dropped a very tiny seed . . ." In this way, your toddler's bite of food becomes an important chapter in the story.

Struggling with food group frustrations? Sneak in a few of these techniques.

Veggies

Dip raw to slightly cooked colorful veggies in sauces or yogurts. Hide veggie purées in mashes, sandwiches, pita pockets, sauces, or soups. Cover veggies with sauces or grated cheese, or flavor them with dill, lemon, honey, olive oil, orange zest, or basil. Grill or roast them to eat alone or on mini-pizzas. Grate them into muffins, pancakes, breads, meatloaves, or salads. (Remember, though—no honey for children less than one year of age.)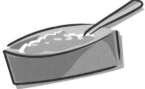

Fruits

Dip fruit shapes in yogurt. Purée fruits to use as dips or spreads or to blend into yogurt smoothies. Bake into muffins, breads, pancakes, meat dishes, or cobblers, or bake them alone. Mix chopped fruit into oatmeal or use it on top of cold cereal. Soften sliced dried fruit in a cup of hot water for fruit stew.

Grains

Substitute wheat flour for half of the white flour in recipes for baked foods. Add two tablespoons of wheat germ, bran, or oat bran into cereals or baked food recipes. Choose wheat pastas, brown rice, and other whole-grain products. Great grains that cook quickly are oats, hominy grits, amaranth, oat bran, quinoa, short grain rice, and bulgur.

Meats and protein

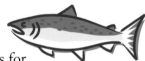

Slice roasted meat or poultry or bake fish sticks for dipping. Chop meats, poultry, or eggs into salads or mixes for sandwiches. Try bean dips, hummus (mashed chickpeas, also known as garbanzo beans), tofu pudding, or nut butters. Use ground beef, poultry, or tempeh (soy-based crumbles) in sauces, quesadillas, soups, or on mini-pizzas.

If your toddler is allergic to wheat, fish, or nuts, see First Course, Allergy Alert, page 18.

11

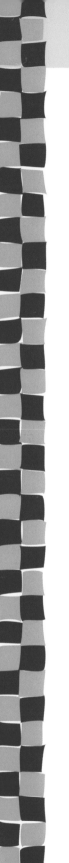

Milk and dairy

Milk is an important source of calcium (see First Course, Allergy Alert, page 18; Beverage Briefs, page 21; and Á la Carte, Notable Nutrients, page 112). If your toddler goes on a milk strike, try alternate calcium sources.

Add plain yogurt to muffins, breads, salads, dips, sauces, smoothies, and as a topping on cereals. Drinkable yogurts such as kefir are also easy options. Look for yogurts with the Live & Active Cultures seal to ensure a supply of friendly, protective bacteria. Some yogurts also contain prebiotics, indigestible fibers that feed the friendly bacteria. See Appendix 2, Shopping Simplicity, page 149.

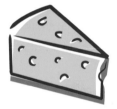 Mix evaporated milk, condensed milk, or nonfat dry milk powder into soups and baked dishes. Cheesy sauces, low-fat cream cheese spreads, cheese strips, melts, or cheese sandwiches are great dairy sources, too!

For vegan toddlers, soy products and other milk substitutes fortified with calcium and vitamin D are good alternative sources of calcium (see Appendix 2, page 149).

Four-star fundamentals

If you only read the end of chapters, then you're in luck, because this section summarizes some important points to help you nurture your toddler's health with good nutrition.

Bistro Basics

Offer toddler-size servings!
Serve one tablespoon of each dish per year of age or about one-quarter of an adult serving at meals and snacks. Toddler stomachs are the size of their fists, so a little goes a long way. If you are in doubt, serve less than what you expect. In one study, three- to five-year-olds who were fed double portion sizes ate 15 to 25 percent more calories than those served proper portions. They can always signal for more! See Á la Carte, Notable Nutrients, page 112, for serving suggestions and nutrient amounts. Check out www.mypyramid.gov for the U.S. government's latest recommendations.

Here are some examples of appropriate toddler-sized portions from the various food groups:

- **Grains:** ½ cup cereal; ½ slice bread
- **Fruit and vegetables:** 2 to 3 tablespoons veggies or fruit
- **Protein:** 1 to 2 ounces meat, poultry, fish, or meat substitutes; 1 egg; 2 tablespoons nut butter; ½ cup beans
- **Dairy:** ½ cup milk or yogurt; 1 ounce cheese

Remember to role model! Your own food preferences directly relate to those your toddler will acquire. You are creating the foundation for your toddler's eating habits in preschool and later in life. I definitely took a hiatus from my mother's healthy role modeling when I was a child to eat French fries and candy, but eventually those nutritious eating habits championed over my little junk food venture.

Communicate with your kitchen crew to establish eating rules for your toddler. Coordinating meals with your family, deciding what foods may enter the house and your toddler's mouth, and practicing mealtime manners send a clear message about acceptable food behaviors to your toddler.

Variety is the spice of life, and food is not excluded! Let your toddler choose from a wide variety, including favorites.

Beverages should follow the main course to prevent your toddler from filling up on fluids. Bistro Bests are water and milk.

Limit desserts and sweets (see First Course, Summing Up Salt, Sugar, and Spice, page 35). My grandfather loved to jokingly respond to our requests for dessert with his family-coined phrase, "Desert the table!"

Encourage self-feeding with fingers or toddler utensils. By two years of age, most toddlers can feed themselves with a spoon. You may need to stand by with a spoon handy to help some food get into the mouth!

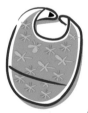

Expect a mess! Poking, smelling, mashing, tossing, and spitting out your recipes are natural stages of development and food acceptance. It doesn't mean that they hate the food! Minimize messes with plastic floor mats, shirt bibs with pockets, plastic grip bowls and suction plates, handy wipes, and a sense of humor! Dogs are fabulous at making floor messes vanish, too!

Routines are reassuring for toddlers. Set regular dining hours for three meals a day (its okay if they only really devour one of them) and two to three snacks a day. At home, designate a specific dining area for snacks and meals. Try to space snacks an hour to an hour and a half before meals.

Bring the family together for meals as often as possible. Today's world of working parents makes it tough, but it's worth it to fit in at least one family meal a week; one a day is even better! Eating together at home provides a sense of structure and security for your toddler. Research shows that eating together leads to a healthier diet with less fat, trans fat, cholesterol, salt, and soda, and more minerals, vitamins, and fiber. If the next available booking for a home family meal isn't until your toddler is a teenager, try picking up or packing a healthy dinner to go and meeting somewhere convenient to work, such as the beach, a park, or a lake for some fun variety.

Create a calm and relaxed dining atmosphere for your toddler. Stress can promote poor appetites. Put off your Table Manners 101 lecture for later and just enjoy your toddler time! Keep TV, newspapers, and toys out of the dining area. Temptations such as these distract toddlers from eating their meal (see Extras, Television Time, page 137).

Power struggles over food are a dead end. Believe it or not, diet improves with less parental control and more of simply providing a variety of healthy food choices. Trust your toddlers when they act or say they are full. "Full" signs are turning the head away, throwing or playing with food, eating more slowly, trying to ditch the high chair, feeding the begging dog, and simply not finishing. Focus on offering many types of nutritious foods, many times.

Food is fuel! Toddlers should be encouraged to eat in response to their body's signal for hunger and to stop eating when they are full. Presenting food as a reward, bribe, or pacifier gives it an alternate meaning and confuses your toddler into thinking that one food is better than another. Bribing your toddler with food may also lead to future obesity problems. Reward good behavior with compliments or hugs.

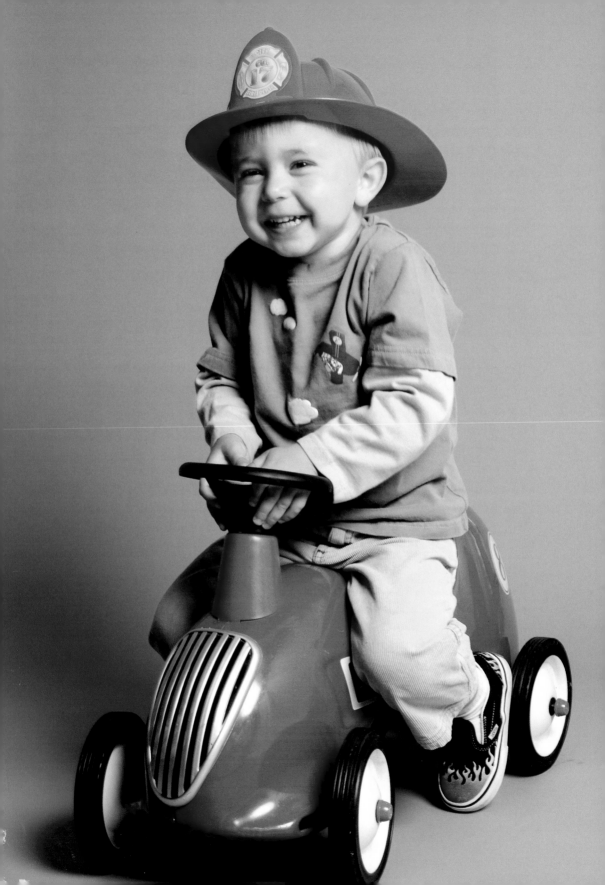

First Course

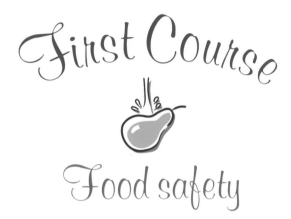

Food safety

Safety is always first when it comes to children, especially regarding food-related issues. As a nutritionist, my worst fear is that parents learn too late about such things as giving their allergy-prone child peanut butter. With access to the correct information, these potential disasters could easily be avoided. I receive many questions from parents about which foods are allergenic or what types of fish are safe to serve to their family. So, here is a quick course on the ins and outs of protecting your toddler from some pitfalls in the world of feeding.

Allergy alert

You survived the first year of eyeing your baby for any reaction after carefully introducing each new food. Keep up the great work as you continue to expand your toddler's palate! If your little one did have a reaction to a certain food, keep it off the menu and discuss with your health care provider when to try reintroducing the food. Food allergies can linger through adolescence, and allergies to peanuts, nuts, and seafood may last a lifetime.

A true food allergy involves an immune-system response to certain foods. Food intolerance reactions do not involve the immune system, but the symptoms and foods that trigger them may overlap with those common to food allergies. The "Bistro Big Eight" below are the most typical allergenic foods.

The Bistro Big Eight allergenic foods

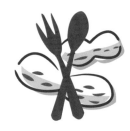

- Eggs
- Milk
- Tree nuts
- Peanuts
- Soy
- Fish
- Shellfish
- Wheat

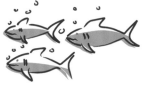

Other foods that may also trigger an allergic or intolerance reaction are berries, especially strawberries, citrus, kiwis, corn products, chocolate, tomatoes, sesame seeds, and mustard seeds.

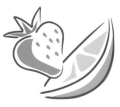

Be aware of how your toddler may present signs of an allergy. Allergic reactions may occur within a few seconds to hours after eating a food, generally after two or three exposures to the food. Physical symptoms of allergy are hives, rash, itching, eczema, facial swelling, wheezing, runny nose, nasal congestion, sneezing, coughing, itchy throat, shortness of breath, asthma, diarrhea, nausea, vomiting, and stomach pain. Hives are the most common allergic reaction.

If you suspect a food allergy, eliminate the questionable food(s) and contact your health care provider. Your toddler may need to be tested for allergies.

Children whose families swim in a genetic pool of allergies (food, environmental, asthma, eczema) have a higher risk of developing food allergies. If your toddler has a parent or sibling with allergies, or has already exhibited eczema or other symptoms of allergy, research suggests that it may be helpful to delay or use extreme caution when you offer allergenic foods. A general guideline for these high-risk children is to monitor or delay serving eggs for the first two years and delay peanuts, tree nuts, shellfish, and fish for the first three years.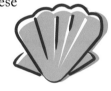

Egg allergies are caused by the egg protein albumin, found mostly in the egg white. Avoid foods containing albumin. Egg substitutes still contain egg protein and should be avoided as well.

Nut allergies are a serious threat and can lead to anaphylactic shock. Do not assume that your toddler is allergic to only one type of nut. Foods that may contain nut remnants are nut oils, nut butters, candy, ice cream, baked goods, and sauces. Be careful when dining out, especially at Chinese, Thai, Mediterranean, and Indian restaurants, where various types of nuts are commonly used. Always ask if the meal contains nuts! Beware of common serving utensils also. Even 1/10,000 of a teaspoon of nuts can trigger an allergic reaction. For a listing of foods recalled due to possible nut contamination, check www.foodallergy.org/alerts.html.

Credit the milk protein casein as the culprit in milk allergies. Avoid foods containing casein or whey (many vegan cheeses still contain casein). Try calcium-fortified soy or rice milks. If your toddler does not tolerate milk 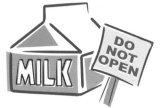 well, but is not truly allergic, he or she may be able to eat yogurts, kefir, or buttermilk without trouble. The bacteria cultures in these products partially break down the milk sugar, lactose, which causes discomfort in some children.

Wheat allergies are caused by the wheat protein gluten. Celiac sprue is a gastrointestinal disorder also caused by a severe reaction to gluten. Avoid foods containing gluten: wheat, barley, rye, oats (unless labeled gluten-free), bulgur, bran, wheat germ, durum flour, einkorn, emmer, graham, kamut, malt, matzo meal, seitan, semolina, spelt, and kasha. For more information on celiac disease, check www.celiac.org.

Try these substitutes for wheat flour: corn flour, cornmeal, rice flour, or potato flour. Soy flour is also an option. It adds extra protein to recipes, but you need to mix it with another type of flour because it does not provide enough structure to baked foods if used alone. These flours also require longer baking times and more leavening (add baking powder) for bread recipes.

Food additives and preservatives such as sodium benzoate, monosodium glutamate (MSG), and artificial flavors and colors may trigger an intolerance reaction, not necessarily the food itself. A small percentage of people may exhibit hives, itching, or wheezing in response to additives. Some studies have linked synthetic food colors with increased irritability or restlessness in susceptible children.

Be a "CLR" (compulsive label reader) on common brands of ketchup, colored drinks, artificial cheese snacks, puddings, cake mixes and icings, and gelatin mixes if you suspect that your toddler is hypersensitive. You may want to try the organic version before giving up on the food. For a complete listing on the safety of food additives, see www.cspinet.org/reports/chemcuisine.htm.

Check www.foodallergy.org for more tips on shopping and cooking around allergies. The Food Allergen Labeling and Consumer Protection Act instructs that food brand labels clearly state whether the product is made with milk, eggs, peanuts, tree nuts, wheat, soy, shellfish, or fish.

Beverage briefs

Now that your toddler has graduated to a sippy cup, what can you put in it? Some parents think that whatever traditional concoction they sipped as toddlers needs to be passed along to their children, but this is not always the case. Here's how to make sure your beverage menu is aboveboard.

Fruit juice

Fruit juice flunks out of the Toddler Bistro diet! Full of sugar and lacking protein, fiber, vitamins, and minerals (unless fortified), it may cause dental

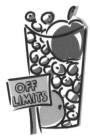

decay, diarrhea, malnutrition, poor appetite, and increases the risk for obesity. Studies show that toddlers who drink a lot of juice tend to drink less milk. Juice also loses out nutritionally to its whole fruit counterparts.

If you choose to offer juice, use only unsweetened, 100 percent juice. Limit serving sizes to ½ cup (4 ounces) diluted with the same amount or more of water, and only serve once a day.

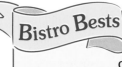

Bistro Bests — **The Toddler Bistro's Best Beverages are milk and water!** Try flavoring water with orange slices or other fresh sliced fruit.

Milk monitor

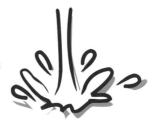

For one- to two-year-olds: Provide full-fat cow's milk or fortified soy milk, 16 to 24 ounces (480 to 720 milliliters) per day. As you wean your toddler from breast milk or formula, you may start substituting these milks when your toddler is around twelve months old. If your toddler sends it back, try mixing the new milk with a little of your breast milk or formula to ease the transition. Keep the full-fat milk flowing until two years of age; toddlers need fat for their developing brains and bodies.

For two- to three-year-olds: Serve 1 percent or 2 percent cow's milk or fortified soy milk, 16 ounces (480 milliliters) per day. Discuss fat-free milk with your health care provider (see Extras, Weight Worries, page 138), if your toddler is overweight or underweight.

Offer milk in half-cup (120-milliliter) servings in a spill-proof cup. Make milk the second course following meals or snacks to encourage eating food first.

Don't overdo it! Milk is very low in iron and interrupts iron absorption. Iron is a mineral that is important for carrying oxygen in the blood. More than 24 ounces per day can cause milk anemia, a condition leading to poor growth, and behavioral and learning problems. Frequent milk drinking also promotes tooth decay.

Soda pop not!

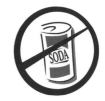

Toddlers should be drinking milk and water. Soda contains empty calories, meaning that its calories are missing vitamins, minerals, and fiber. Soda (sugar and sugar-free) displaces better beverages like milk from toddler diets, can compromise the immune system, dehydrate, interfere with nutrient absorption, and contribute to obesity.

Water wise

Train your toddler early to select water from the menu. This refreshment is popular when served in fun cups and can be flavored with slices of orange or other fresh fruit. Have refills available in hot weather and during highly active times. Watch for signs of dehydration: dark urine in small amounts, thirst, flushed appearance, headache, fever,

> **Bistro Believe It or Not**
>
> In 1945, Americans drank four times more milk than soda. In 1997, they drank two and a half times more soda than milk! Research shows that 72 percent of two- to three-year-olds are drinking about one cup of soda every day.

tiredness, dry mouth, or fast breathing. Vomiting and diarrhea can dehydrate as well. Contact your health care provider in this situation for advice on electrolyte repletion.

If you use bottled water, check your bottled water brand for National Sanitation Foundation–International (NSF) certification, or call 800-NSF-MARK (you get to speak with a human!). Visit online at www.nsf.org. Also check to see if your brand belongs to the International Bottled Water Association through www.epa.gov/safewater.

If you use tap water, heavy metals and contaminants may be present. To test your tap water, find certified labs by calling the Safe Drinking Water Hotline (800) 426-4791.

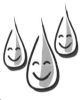

Your drinking water should contain less then three parts per billion (ppb) of lead. You can order a household water test kit for $17 from Clean Water Lead Testing Inc. Go to: www.leadtesting.org/orderonline.htm.

You may find that a filtering system works for you. Companies like Brita claim to remove 98 to 99 percent of lead, cadmium, mercury, and chloride, while 95 percent of the fluoride remains.

If you serve tap water and it contains less than 0.3 parts per million of fluoride, or if you serve unfluoridated bottled water, your toddler may need a fluoride supplement. The adequate intake (AI) for children one to three years of age is 0.7 milligrams per day. To find out about the fluoride content in your community water, call your local public works department or check My Water's Fluoride at http://apps.nccd.cdc.gov/MWF/Index.asp. Consult your health care provider or pediatric dentist about whether to offer a supplement. Fluoride is essential in building strong teeth and bones.

Bug basics

We are talking about food contamination by bacteria (*Staphylococcus A, Listeria, Salmonella, E. coli*), virus (hepatitis A), and parasites (*Giardia*)! These are bugs that toddlers' immature immune systems are not prepared to tackle. Symptoms are diarrhea, stiff neck, fever, cramps, and headache.

Forbidden foods

Although many of the following foods are healthy and delicious, toddlers are more susceptible to the contaminants that they occasionally contain. Keep these foods out of your toddler's reach for the first three years.

- **Alfalfa sprouts:** Raw sprouts may contain *Salmonella*, *E. coli*, and the canavanine toxin.

- **Soft, unpasteurized cheeses:** Glorious gourmet cheeses such as Brie, feta, blue-veined, Camembert, Mexican-style (queso blanco, queso fresco, queso de crea, panela, asadero), and goat cheese may contain *Listeria*.

- **Hot dogs and packaged deli meats:** Besides being not very nutritious, these meats may contain *Listeria* bacteria. Freshly sliced meat from the deli is okay.

- **Raw fish:** Still no sushi for your toddler! Raw fish can carry the hepatitis A virus, bacteria, and parasites.

- **Raw or partially cooked eggs:** Super yummy, but cookie dough, batters, eggnog, Caesar dressing, hollandaise sauce, homemade ice cream, and chocolate mousse are off-limits to toddlers. These foods may contain bacteria or parasites.

- **Unpasteurized milk, juice, or cider:** We need pasteurization to wipe out bacteria like *Listeria*!

Bug-proofing the Bistro

Set your refrigerator temperature for 40°F (5°C) to protect the foods inside from spoiling. Practice safe food storage with the following guidelines:

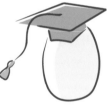

- **Eggs:** Store raw, in shells, for up to three weeks; store hard-boiled eggs for one week.

- **Fish and meat:** Refrigerate for two days, then freeze.

- **Vegetables:** Refrigerate for two to five days.

- **Cooked foods:** Refrigerate for three days and do not leave out at room temperature for more than two hours.

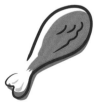

- Marinate meats and fish in the fridge, not at room temperature, and toss the used marinade.

- Weird-smelling foods, moldy parts of cheeses, moldy breads, unopened cans with dents or bulges, and punctured packaged foods are all trash-worthy!

- For foods in the freezer, set your freezer temperature for 0°F (−18°C). Defrost foods in a plastic bag in the fridge, in cold water (½ hour per pound), or in the microwave on the defrost setting. Don't defrost at room temperature. Cook defrosted meats or fish immediately.

Cooking clues

Now that you know how to store food, how do you cook it? I know it seems tedious, but these clean culinary techniques are important to prevent bugs from setting up camp where they don't belong.

Wash your hands religiously with soap and warm water for at least twenty seconds before and after contact with food, especially raw meats and fish.

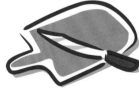

Use separate cutting boards and knives: one for raw meats and fish and another for cooked foods, fruits, and veggies. Sanitize non-wood boards in the dishwasher. For wooden boards, scrub with hot, soapy water or bleach. Replace wooden boards if they are deeply nicked.

Sponges and kitchen cloths or towels should not be used with raw meats and fish. Wash them often. Microwave sponges for thirty to sixty seconds or throw them in the dishwasher to kill bugs. Use disposable paper towels for meat and fish juice spills.

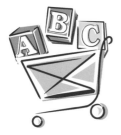

Shopping suggestions

Check expiration dates. Put raw meats in bags and keep them separate from produce. Add the cold and frozen foods to your cart last at the store. Freeze or refrigerate foods quickly when you are back home.

Packing for picnics

Transport foods in a cooler with freezer packs and place it in a shady area or cover it with a towel once you reach your picnic spot. One trick is to prepare sandwiches the night before and refrigerate them overnight so that they stay colder in transit. If your toddler thinks that the lake or creek water is perfect for sippy cup refills, just say no! The consequences from children drinking contaminated water are not fun for moms.

Bistro Basics for a grime-free toddler

Keep diaper wipes in the car and in the stroller to clean hands and faces. Alcohol wipes are convenient for sanitizing shopping carts, restaurant tables, or high chairs. Laundry wipes help remove clothes stains immediately.

Cool the caffeine

It's definitely a little early for a sippy cup o' joe every morning! Caffeine is a diuretic and an artificial stimulant that triggers the adrenal glands to release adrenalin, making for a hyper toddler. Caffeine content is high in sodas, coffee, tea, and cold and headache medications. Lesser amounts of caffeine are found in chocolate. Two colas for a toddler equal eight cups of coffee for an adult!

Choking checks

Avoid nuts, seeds, popcorn, chips, pretzels, vegetable and fruit skins, whole raw apples and carrots, whole green beans, small dried fruits, whole grapes and cherries, whole olives, berries, melon balls, tough or big pieces of meat, hot dogs, hard cookies and biscuits, globs of peanut butter and nut butters, pickles, and BIG BITES.

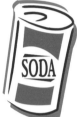

Toddler diners should be seated when eating and should not giggle or talk while chewing.

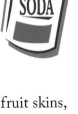

Cook fruits and veggies according to how many teeth your toddler has, and supervise your toddler during dining!

Fishy fish

Seafood is a favorite in the nutrition world for its fabulous health benefits, wide range of choices, and tastes that appeal to most people, even selective toddlers. A few of our aquatic friends, however, are best left in the water due to potentially harmful contaminants.

Crustacean clues

Shellfish such as shrimp, crab, lobster, mussels, scallops, oysters, clams, crayfish, etc. are very allergenic (see Allergy Alert, page 18). Although many of these shelled sea dwellers are excellent sources of protein and minerals, they can trigger allergies in sensitive children. Hold off on shellfish for your toddler until after his or her first two birthdays.

Fish and the mercury menace

Avoid swordfish, shark, tuna (including ahi steaks), gold or white snapper, king mackerel, marlin, bluefish, wild striped bass, walleye, and tilefish. Do not serve from birth to two years of age.

These predator fish can store dangerous levels of mercury that accumulate in the body if they are eaten regularly. The older, larger fish contain the highest amounts. Mercury poisoning in humans causes potential heart damage, delayed development, nerve disorders, and mental retardation. Because the first two years of life are crucial for brain development, it is important to choose low-contaminant fish for your toddlers. For a complete list of mercury content in fish, see http://www.fda.gov/Food/FoodSafety/Product-SpecificInformation/Seafood/FoodbornePathogensContaminants/Methylmercury/ucm115644.htm.

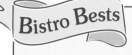

Bistro Best choices for fish feasts
Pacific sole or flounder, wild salmon (see farmed salmon on page 31), farmed Arctic char, U.S. tilapia, catfish, turbot, herring, mahi-mahi, sardines, farmed striped bass, red snapper, pollock, rainbow trout, Pacific halibut, and sablefish.

Check fish advisories before serving fish caught recreationally by family or friends from lakes, rivers, or the ocean. Uncle Joe's prized catch that he delivers from his annual fishing expedition may not be safe for children.

See www.edf.org and www.epa.gov/waterscience/fish for a listing of fish advisories. Look for "Seafood Safe" labels in supermarkets and restaurants.

Bistro Basics

Best choice for tuna? Use canned, chunk-light skipjack tuna. Canned white albacore tuna contains higher levels of mercury. The Federal Drug Administration (FDA) and Environmental Protection Agency (EPA) advise women who are pregnant, nursing, or may become pregnant, and children under age twelve that they may eat up to 12 ounces of low-mercury fish per week. Six of those ounces may be white albacore tuna. Due to conflicting research on mercury levels in canned tuna, however, it may be prudent to completely avoid this selection. If you purchase tuna, choose canned light tuna, typically prepared from smaller fish with lower mercury levels. Try substituting canned wild salmon for a similar-tasting yet safer dish, and vary the fish on the menu.

The scoop on salmon

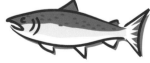

For farmed salmon, serve one serving per month (two per month if served broiled or grilled). It's okay to serve wild salmon twice per week.

To farm or not to farm? This is the question! Being at the top of the food chain, we care that our favorite fish eat healthy foods. Wild salmon feast on deep-ocean krill, green algae, and other small fish. Farmed salmon are fed concentrated fish meal and fish oil derived from waters closer to shore that may be contaminated with carcinogenic polychlorinated biphenyls (PCBs) and dioxins. The fish oil makes salmon grow faster but also houses these fat-loving toxins. A recent study* found that farmed salmon has seven times more PCBs and dioxins than wild salmon. The highest levels were found in Scottish and Northern European farmed salmon, which account for only 7 percent of U.S. salmon.

Salmon farmers are working to clean up their fish food, but until they do, follow these Bistro Basics:

- Select a healthy variety of fish. Catfish and trout are less contaminated farmed fish containing good sources of omega-3 oil. Try to buy salmon wild or from organic farms. Organic fish encounter fewer pesticides, eat fish trimmings fit for humans, and live in less-crowded pens. Trim fat (chemicals accumulate in fat) and score the fish, then broil or grill so that the juice drips off. You will still get plenty of the healthy omega-3 fish oil. Remove the skin before eating.

- Ask at restaurants if the fish is wild. All Alaskan salmon is wild, as is most canned salmon (a good calcium source, too). The best wild salmon varieties are coho, pink, and chum.

---

*Hites, et al. Global Assessment of Organic Contaminants in Farmed Salmon. *Science* 303 (January 9, 2004).

- Don't be scared out of the water! The omega-3 oils in ANY salmon, trout, or other fish provide us with much greater benefits, for cardiovascular and developmental health, than risks, with their relatively minimal risk of cancer.

- Check www.eatwellguide.org for organic food delivery or stores near you.

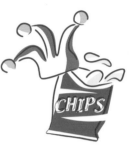

Foolish fats

Certain fats are potentially harmful for growing toddlers' brains and bodies. The following are some fats to pass on.

Trans fats

Breast-feeding moms, all toddlers, and everyone else should completely avoid or at least minimize eating this type of fat. Partially hydrogenated trans fats are commercially altered fats that make oils more stable and increase food's shelf life. They are used in products

Bistro Basics

Be a "CLR" (compulsive label reader). The good news is that all food labels are required to list trans fats. Avoid products with "partially hydrogenated oil" or "trans fat" in the contents. Product labels may list "zero trans fats" if they have less than half a gram of trans fats per serving, so scan ingredient lists to make sure that trans fats are not slipping in under the radar.

such as bakery foods, breads, snacks, and margarines. They contribute to the risk for diabetes and heart disease and interfere with growth and development.

Low-fat and fat-free products

Unless special circumstances exist (see Extras, Weight Worries, page 138), children under the age of two need full-fat foods and beverages to support healthy brain and body development. After two years of age, you may begin to substitute low-fat products for their full-fat counterparts.

Macrobiotic diets

This diet is a no-no for toddlers! Toddlers have small appetites and small stomachs and go through picky stages, and their diet needs to offer plenty of energy and nutrients. Macrobiotic diets consist mainly of whole grains, produce, and a little fish, resulting in a diet low in calories, protein, fat, vitamins, and minerals, thus jeopardizing normal growth. These diets can lead to "failure to thrive" in young children.

Meats to miss

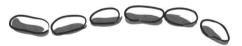

Avoid bacon, sausages, hot dogs, cured meats, and packaged deli meats. (Freshly sliced meats from the deli are okay.) Besides being high in fat and salt, they contain sodium nitrite, a preservative that can be cancer causing when these meats are cooked at high temperatures and also when sodium nitrite reacts with chemicals in the stomach. Recent data show that 27 percent of toddlers are eating hot dogs, bacon, and sausage—not a healthy diet!

Look for healthier options such as turkey or soy-based sausage or hot dogs, and be a "CLR" (compulsive label reader) for nitrites or nitrates on labels. See Appendix 2, Shopping Simplicity, page 149, for some healthy brands.

Slipping in the sippy cup

If you haven't done so already, the time between twelve and eighteen months is when you should lose the bottle and start introducing milk in a sippy cup at meals and snacks. To encourage eating solid food, first banish the bottle at meals, and bottle feed or breast feed only at snacks and bedtime.

Typically, the bedtime bottle is the last to go. Try serving a cup of milk after dinner and substitute water for milk in the bedtime bottle. Eventually, the bottle attraction will fade. Although it's okay if your toddler still asks for the bottle at two years of age, the longer you wait to wean your child from the bottle, the harder it gets.

Never let toddlers go to sleep with the bottle! Constant sucking may affect palate formation and speech, and overexposure to the sugar in milk can cause tooth decay.

Summing up salt, sugar, and spice

We love to experiment with the flavor of our food, and tasting our creations is part of what makes eating so much fun. But . . . keep these health tips in mind for your toddler tasters.

Skip the salt

We get plenty naturally. Use half the salt (iodized) called for in recipes, choose low-salt brand foods (fast food and processed foods are salt magnets), and keep the shaker off the table!

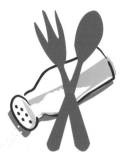

Are sugar and spice really so nice?

Spices should be introduced slowly. Toddlers have more taste buds than adults, increasing their sensitivity to flavors. Depending on family or cultural customs, toddlers' preferences for spices will vary.

Toddlers will get sugar one way or the other, so your job is to moderate how much and how often. Research has shown that early introduction to sugary foods encourages sugar cravings as adults. Simple sugars such as those in soda, candy, cookies, sugary cereals, and fruit drinks spike blood sugar, trigger more sugar cravings, and may compromise the immune system. Filling up on sugary foods also increases the chance for diarrhea and dental decay, and it displaces healthier menu selections.

If you do have sugar on the menu, serve it with a balanced meal to even out energy levels and to avoid sugar "burnout" (low energy).

Bistro Basics for supervising sugar
Keep sugar out of the house, and "cupboard" your sweet cravings! If you must, sneak a little chocolate from your stash during naptime. You are your toddler's role model for nutrition.

Don't make too big a deal out of the occasional dessert, because your toddler might get the idea that desserts are better than other foods. On birthdays, the whole day is special, not just the cake!

Cut the sugar in recipes by one quarter to one third.

Be a "CLR" (compulsive label reader) for sugar imposters like high fructose corn syrup (HFCS), dextrose, sucrose, and modified food starch when they are listed in the top three or four ingredients. Toddlers in search of sweets may be tyrants, but set your sugar rules and stay strong!

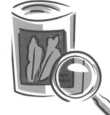

Avoid artificial sweeteners. Unless special circumstances such as diabetes exist, there is no need for sugar substitutes in your toddler's diet. Use a little of the real thing.

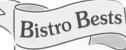

Bistro Bests for sweeteners
Try sweet-tasting and less refined sugars like 100 percent fruit purées (less effect on raising blood sugar), dark honey (after the toddler is one year old), dark maple syrup, blackstrap molasses, or cinnamon, a spice that research indicates may help even out blood sugar levels.

Shopping smarts

Grocery shopping can be quite overwhelming, especially with your toddler riding along in the shopping cart. You have to keep your eye on your little Houdini, who is trying to wiggle out of the cart, and at the same time keep him or her distracted from wanting every item in the junk food aisle. My guess is that you may not be able to study every food label and that you would probably prefer to enter and exit the grocery store as quickly as possible. I have asked parents whether they want general guidelines regarding what to look for at the market, or if they simply want to be told which are the best brands to buy. The majority answered, "Just tell us what to buy!"

I decided to do both. Keep in mind that there are thousands of brands out there and they are constantly evolving. Some companies offer wonderful products, but they are only distributed regionally. It is nearly impossible to list all of the good brands, so here's some help for narrowing your food search. The following tips offer general guidelines on how to navigate the grocery maze and choose healthy foods. For some specific brand suggestions, visit Appendix 2, Shopping Simplicity, page 149.

Shopping trip tips

For easy shopping, make your list according to the aisles in your favorite market. Keep your list in an accessible spot, like on the refrigerator, so that you can add to it as the thought pops into your head. You'll forget two seconds later!

Look for the appropriate age range on the labels of children's food brands.

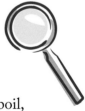

Opt for organic! Check the frozen section for organic fruits and veggies. They are less expensive and will not spoil, which means that they can be used as needed.

Add meats, fish, and frozen foods to your cart last to maximize freshness.

Buy whole-fat dairy items for your baby through two years of age.

Shop for extra frozen favorites to store with grandparents or anywhere you visit frequently.

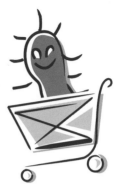

Keep a small antiseptic spray handy for dirty grocery carts that your baby may want to taste!

Point out different colors and shapes of fruits and vegetables to your toddler and talk about why they are healthy.

Practice your "CLR" (compulsive label reader) skills, and do your best to avoid the following ingredients:

- Trans fats (partially hydrogenated fats)
- Hydrogenated oils, lard, palm kernel oil, coconut oils, shortening, and beef tallow (in the top three ingredients)
- Saturated fat (more than 3 grams per serving)
- Sodium (more than 140 milligrams per serving)
- Sugar, high fructose corn syrup (HFCS), fructose, honey, glucose, sucrose (in the top three ingredients)
- Food additives: nitrates, nitrites, sulfites, artificial flavoring or coloring

If your toddler has food allergies, check labels to see if the food contains any allergy-related ingredient. Albumin (egg), casein (milk), and gluten (wheat) are allergenic proteins from foods. The Food Allergen Consumer Protection Act instructs companies to clearly list on food labels whether the product is made with milk, eggs, peanuts, tree nuts, wheat, soy, shellfish, or fish.

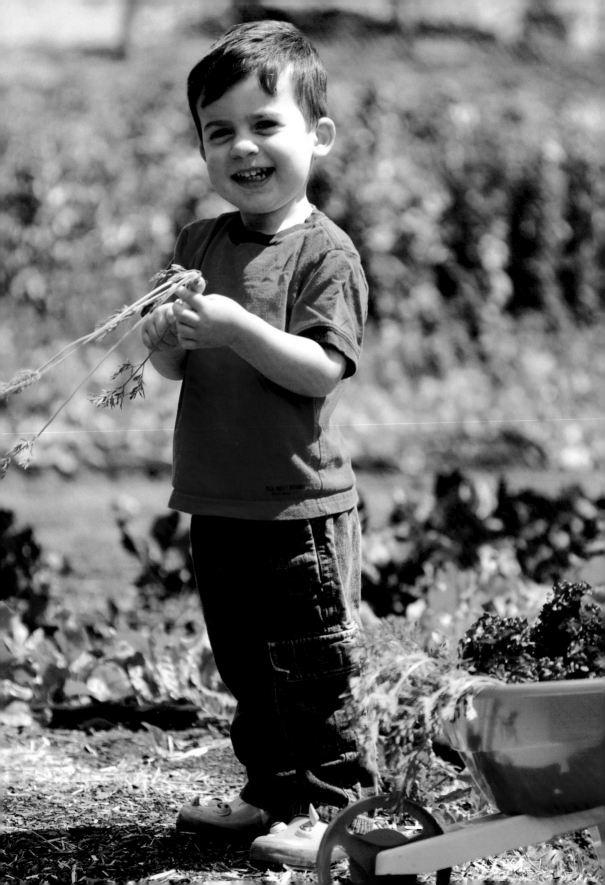

Second Course

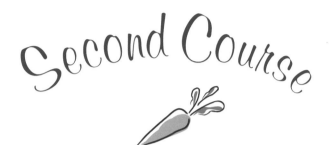

Family environmental health

In many ways, humans live much more removed from the natural environment than most other animals, except for my dog, who could not survive for a second in nature without his toys and treats! This is a consequence of modern living, making our lives very convenient, yet also exposing us to potentially harmful toxic residues from our man-made products and technologies.

Children exposed to chemical toxins during crucial stages of development may be more vulnerable to their effects than adults. It is important to adopt some basic habits like storing cleaning products in a cupboard out of toddler's reach and keeping a list of emergency numbers (Poison Control, doctor, neighbor) on an inside door of a kitchen cabinet for you and care providers.

Other unhealthy environmental substances that we encounter regularly are less obvious. Scientific research has already led to government bans on some toxins, and studies continue to reveal others that may pose significant health threats. In the meantime, it is good practice to minimize your family's contact with these unwelcome invaders.

Good grilling

Contact between fat in foods and the flame, hot coals, or your grill's heating element causes carcinogenic chemicals called heterocyclic amines (HCAs) to form on the food. Everyone loves a good barbeque, but follow some Bistro Basics for safe grilling:

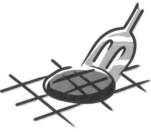

- **Avoid charring foods. Cut off and toss the burned parts.**

- **Half-bake food in the oven, then finish it on the grill.**

- **Try an herbed marinade. Some research suggests that the natural antioxidants in herbs decrease the amount of HCAs formed during grilling.**

Keeping out the lead

Lead poisoning can cause learning disabilities and diminished attention span in children. Lead-based paint may be a problem in homes built before 1978 and is even more of a threat in pre-1946 homes. Double-check painted toys, windowsills, trim work, and doorways. Water pipes may contain lead (see First Course, Beverage Briefs, page 21). Lastly, love your lead crystal all you want, but don't store food in it! Avoid storing food in ceramic dishes as well.

Check www.epa.gov/lead or call the National Lead Information Center, (800) 424-LEAD.

Pesticide perils

If only they just killed bugs. Unfortunately, pesticides may also block toddlers' ability to absorb nutrients from foods, which interferes with normal weight gain and brain development. Pesticides have also been shown to decrease the normal vitamin and mineral content of some fruits and vegetables.

Toddlers are more vulnerable to these dangers for several reasons:

- Toddlers' organ systems aren't fully developed to defend against and filter and excrete toxic chemicals.

- Toddlers eat a more limited diet than adults.

- Toddlers eat and drink more in proportion to their body weight than adults.

- Toddlers explore anything within reach with their hands and mouths.

- According to the National Academy of Sciences, 50 percent of lifetime pesticide exposure occurs during the first five years of life.

So what's a parent to do? Here are some easy kitchen basics to help get rid of residues from your produce.

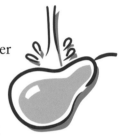

Wash and scrub all fruits and veggies using warm water and a little liquid dish soap. Don't forget to wash produce with rinds, like cantaloupes and oranges, because your cutting knife transfers pesticides and bacteria into the fruit. Remove outer leaves and break apart broccoli or cauliflower before washing.

- Serve a wide variety of produce.
- Buy seasonally or locally grown foods (less spraying and wax coating).
- Trim fats from meat, poultry, and fish (fatty tissue attracts chemicals).
- Wash can lids before opening them.

Bistro Bests

Whenever you can, opt for organic! Look for the USDA 100 Percent Certified Organic seal on foods. It means that no artificial ingredients or preservatives are present and that foods are grown without conventional pesticides, antibiotics, hormones, irradiation, or genetically modified foods. Organic foods have also been found to contain more nutrients than regular produce.

Organic foods may take up a chunk of your income, so spend selectively on the items below and also check for less costly frozen organic brands.

Save some grocery money by buying conventionally grown produce from the Conventional Keepers foods, and spend a little extra on organically grown produce from the foods in the Dirty Dozen.

The Dirty Dozen	Conventional Keepers
(highest pesticide residues)	(lowest pesticide residues)
Apples	Asparagus
Bell peppers	Avocados
Celery	Bananas
Cherries	Broccoli
Imported grapes	Cauliflower
Peaches	Kiwis
Pears	Mangos
Potatoes	Onions
Nectarines	Papayas
Red raspberries	Pineapples
Spinach	Sweet corn
Strawberries	Sweet peas

The more we demand organic foods, the more affordable they become. Check www.consumersunion.org for updates on pesticide residues in food. To find organic food stores near you or to order organic food for delivery, check www.eatwellguide.org or www.iatp.org.

Plastics in the news

Plastic materials pervade our daily lives through many different products or devices. They are quite useful in supporting structure and durability in various forms of packaging. However, some of their chemical components are like an antivitamin if they migrate into our bodies.

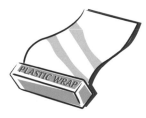

Plastic wraps

Toddlers are vulnerable to certain chemicals (dioxins and DEHA) found in some plastic wraps, which may disrupt their normal hormone, immune, cognitive, and growth development. These chemical plasticizers leach from plastic wrap into fatty and acidic foods, especially in the presence of heat and light.

Bistro Basics

Leave an inch or more space between food and plastic wrap when storing food in the refrigerator or heating it in the microwave.

Plastics and the microwave

We all know we can't microwave with metal, but from there things get a little confusing. Here is a list of safe materials for the microwave:

- Corningware
- Microwave-safe glass
- Microwave cooking bags
- White paper towels
- Wax paper
- Parchment paper

Never microwave food in take-out containers, margarine tubs, plastic storage bags, grocery bags, or used microwave dinner containers. Put frozen meals in microwave-safe dishes to defrost them.

Check www.fsis.usda.gov/factsheets/cooking_safely_in_ the_microwave/index.asp.

Plastics and food preservation

Store leftovers in glass containers or baggies and repackage plastic-wrapped store-bought foods and take-out foods packaged in Styrofoam containers when you get home. And throw away those old plastic containers!

Bisphenol A (BPA) plastic containers

Scientists are concerned about studies indicating that this chemical compound may interfere with human hormone and nervous system functions and increase the risk for certain cancers. They question the safety of BPA exposure, especially in infants and children during important stages of development.

Plastic food-storage containers, beverage containers, and the linings of some cans may contain BPA. Some manufacturers have removed BPA from their products, but not all of them, so here I go again with my label-reading lecture!

Check that your toddler's sippy cup, water bottles, food-storage containers, and canned foods are BPA-free. Food packaged in pouches, cardboard cartons, or glass is a safer alternative. For more information, see www.cspinet.org/nah/bpa.html and www.ewg.org.

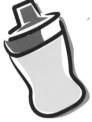

Stove-top and oven cookware smarts

If your favorite cooking methods include using the stove top or oven regularly, you need reliable cookware that distributes heat evenly and also does not risk releasing toxic chemicals into your food or the air. Some materials used in nonstick coatings are potentially harmful, as are unlined pots and pans fashioned from standard metals such as aluminum and copper.

Stock your kitchen with choices from this list of Bistro Best stove-top and oven cookware:

- **Anodized aluminum**
- **Cast iron** (a good choice especially for vegans, to add extra iron into cooked foods)
- **Stainless steel**
- **Lined copper**
- **Silicone** (filler-free)
- **Heatproof glass**

Avoid cooking foods on extremely high heat if you use pots and pans with nonstick coating. Get rid of chipped or flaking pots and pans. Now you have a great excuse to shop for the Chef!

Smoke signals

Tobacco smoke, secondhand smoke, and environmental smoke put your child at risk for respiratory infections, ear infections, asthma, decreased lung function, pneumonia, and cancer.

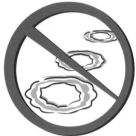

Follow these Bistro Basics to keep your toddler clear of smoke. If you smoke, do it outside. Change your clothes when you come back inside. Secondhand smoke lingers on furniture and clothes and poses the same health risks as breathing in smoke directly. Ask relatives and guests who smoke to step outside.

Check www.epa.gov/smokefree/and www.cdc.gov.

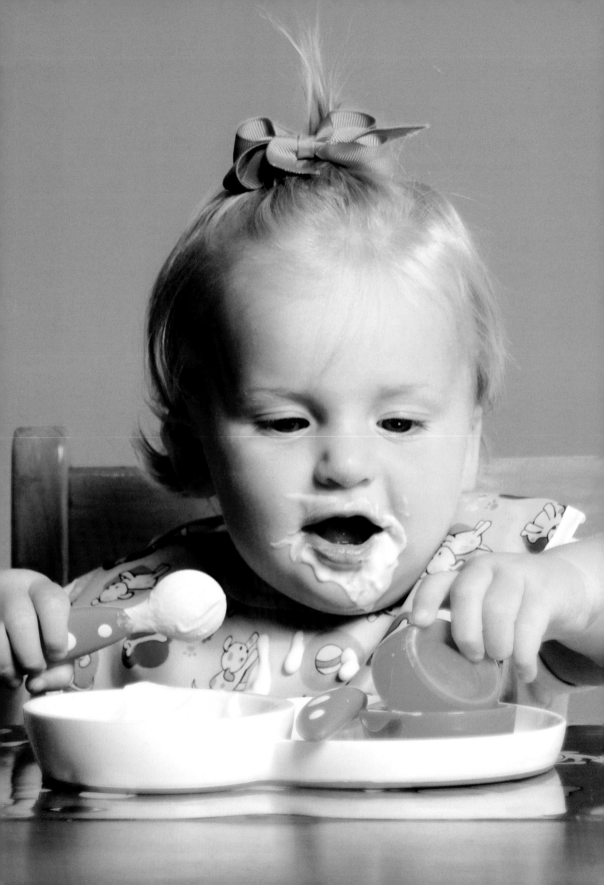

Entrées

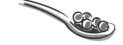

In the early years, from ages one to three

One to three years old is a fun stage when you get to introduce many new foods. Whether you plan to cook every meal at home or purchase foods at the store, your goal should be to put the baby food away and start offering your toddler kid-friendly versions of foods from the family meal. You may still purée some foods if necessary; however, most toddlers have teeth at this age and should start adjusting to new textures other than smooth baby purées. Some toddlers become dependent on purées if parents continue offering them beyond the first year.

Entrées

I know that it is easier to make recipes liked by the whole family, not just your toddler, so each recipe in this section has been tasted by toddlers to teens and beyond. If your toddler wants breakfast for dinner or dinner for breakfast, that is fine. As long as the meal offers healthy food group choices, it's all good. All entrées are interchangeable depending upon the taste and preference of your esteemed Toddler Bistro patrons!

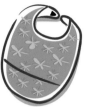

Daily nutrient needs for one- to two-year-olds
This table is simply a guide to recommended daily dietary intakes for those inquiring minds that want to know. It is not set in stone, so no worries!

Pounds	Calories	Protein(g)	Fat(g)	Carbs(g)	Fiber(g)
15	530	8	26	59	7
20	730	10	37	82	7
25	930	12	47	105	7
30	1,130	15	57	128	7
35	1,340	17	67	150	7
40	1,540	20	77	173	7

Your toddler should gain a little less than his or her birth weight and grow about two to three inches this year. Also expect more teeth and first molars. Growth spurts are sporadic, but usually growth patterns normalize by two years of age. Your health care provider will help you monitor your toddler's growth.

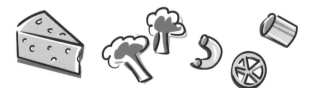

Daily nutrient needs for two- to three-year-olds
This table is the same as the table for one- to two-year-olds, except now fat is only 30 percent of calories and fiber is increased.

Pounds	Calories	Protein(g)	Fat(g)	Carbs(g)	Fiber(g)
20	730	8	24	82	8
25	930	10	31	105	8
30	1,130	15	38	128	8
35	1,340	17	45	150	8
40	1,540	20	51	173	8
45	1,740	22	58	196	8

Your toddler should gain around five pounds, grow a couple of inches, and cut second molars this year. Your health care provider will help you monitor your toddler's growth.

Bravo for breakfast!

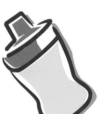

Even if your toddler chooses 5 A.M. as the perfect time to start the day, studies show that toddlers who eat breakfast are better behaved, have increased attention spans, have better problem-solving skills, have boosted metabolisms, and have a lower risk for obesity than those who skip this meal. No time to cook? See Appendix 2, Shopping Simplicity, page 149, for a shortcut to brand suggestions. Anyone at any age can get stuck in a rut when it comes to creative, nutritious, and easy breakfasts. There is life after rice cereal, so have fun trying some of these toddler-tested yummy meals to start the day! All Toddler Bistro breakfasts include a complimentary sippy cup of milk.

Swiss granola
MAKES A SINGLE SERVING

- ½ cup plain yogurt
- ½ cup low-sugar dry cereal
- 1 teaspoon 100 percent fruit preserves

In a toddler dish, spoon half of the yogurt, then half of the cereal, the preserves, the rest of the yogurt, and the rest of the cereal. Top with a sprinkle of blueberries or sliced bananas. *(See photo on opposite page.)*

Sooo good pumpkin pancakes
MAKES 4 SERVINGS

- ½ cup cornmeal
- ½ cup all-purpose flour
- ¼ teaspoon ginger
- ½ teaspoon cinnamon
- 1 pinch nutmeg
- 1 teaspoon baking powder
- Dash of salt
- ¼ cup packed brown sugar
- 1 teaspoon orange zest
- ½ cup peeled, chopped apples, raisins, or walnuts
- ½ cup puréed pumpkin
- ⅓ cup milk
- 1 egg

Sift dry ingredients together except for the sugar. Mix in the sugar along with the rest of the ingredients. Pour 2 to 3 tablespoons of batter per pancake onto a hot, oiled griddle and cook through on both sides. Serve with a little maple syrup, fresh fruit, or yogurt.

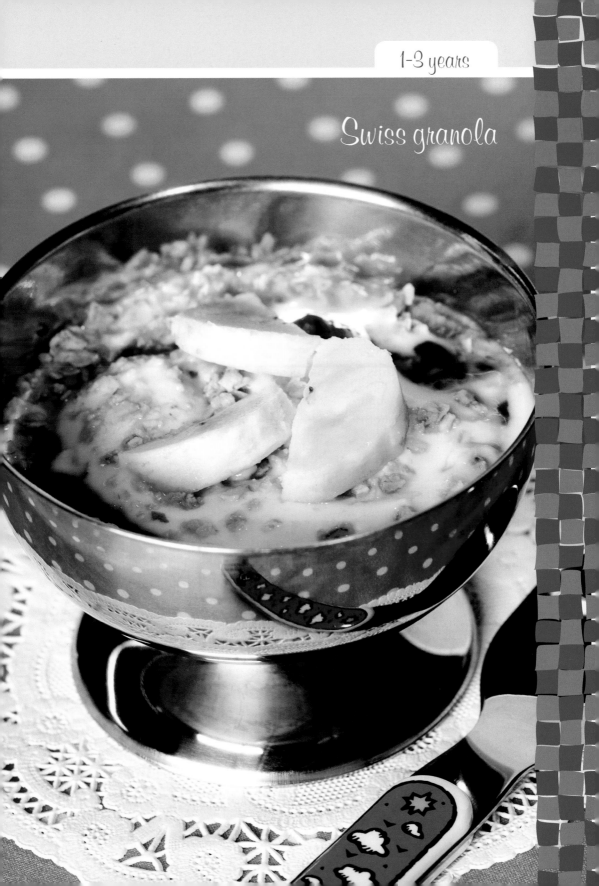

Swiss granola

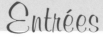
Gramma Joanie's cottage cakes

**MAKES APPROXIMATELY
20 MINI-CAKES**

- ¼ cup all-purpose flour
- 1½ teaspoons canola oil
- 3 eggs
- 1 cup cottage cheese

Mix together all ingredients, then pour in heaping tablespoons onto a hot, oiled griddle. Cook on both sides until golden. Top with grated cheddar cheese, applesauce, maple syrup, or fruit spread. *(See photo on opposite page.)*

Orange-oat muffins

MAKES APPROXIMATELY ONE DOZEN MUFFINS

- ½ cup plain yogurt
- ¼ cup canola oil
- 2 egg whites
- ½ cup maple syrup
- 1 cup whole wheat or oat bran flour
- ½ cup rolled oats
- 1 cup all-purpose flour
- 2 teaspoons baking powder
- 1 teaspoon cinnamon
- 1 large apple, peeled and chopped
- 2 teaspoons orange zest
- ½ cup raisins

Whisk together the wet ingredients. Mix in the dry ingredients and add the fruit. Line or oil a regular-sized muffin tin. Pour the mixture into the cups almost to the top. Bake at 400° F for 20 to 25 minutes.

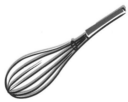

Gramma Joanie's cottage cakes

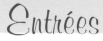

Sunday egg scramble

MAKES 3–4 SERVINGS

- 4 eggs
- ¼ cup milk
- 2 teaspoons canola oil or cooking spray
- ½ cup chopped broccoli
- ½ cup chopped red bell pepper
- ½ cup chopped sweet onion
- ½ cup grated cheese

Beat the eggs with milk. Sauté the veggies in oil, then add the egg mixture and cheese. For a heartier scramble, stir in some sliced cooked poultry sausage, chopped cooked meat, or shredded cooked potatoes. Serve with sliced fruit. Vegan substitutions are 8 ounces of firm tofu, vegan sausage, and ½ cup soy cheese. Tofu needs 3 to 4 minutes to cook.

Refrigerator raisin bran muffins

MAKES APPROXIMATELY TWO DOZEN MUFFINS

- 2½ cups raisin bran
- ½ cup packed brown sugar
- 1 cup whole wheat flour
- 1½ cups all-purpose flour
- 2½ teaspoons baking soda
- 1 teaspoon salt
- 2 eggs
- ½ cup canola oil
- 2 cups buttermilk

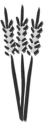

Mix the raisin bran, sugar, flour, soda, and salt in a large mixing bowl. Add the eggs, oil, and buttermilk. Store in a covered container in the refrigerator and use as desired. Let the batter reach room temperature before baking. Use vegetable cooking spray or line a regular-sized muffin tin. Fill cups two-thirds full and bake at 400° F for 15 to 20 minutes.

Tofu French toast

MAKES 6 SERVINGS

- 8 ounces silken tofu
- ½ cup plain soy milk
- 1 tablespoon maple syrup
- ¼ teaspoon nutmeg
- ½ teaspoon cinnamon
- 6 or more slices whole-grain bread, cut diagonally or into fun shapes

Blend all ingredients except for the bread. Dip the bread slices into the mixture and cook in an oiled skillet on medium-high heat on both sides until browned. Serve with 100 percent fruit purées.

Traditional French toast

MAKES 6 SERVINGS

- 1 egg
- 1 cup milk
- ½ teaspoon vanilla
- 1 teaspoon each of cinnamon, nutmeg, and salt
- 6 or more slices whole-grain bread, sliced diagonally or cut into fun shapes

Whisk together the egg, milk, vanilla, and spices. Dip the bread slices in the mixture and place in oiled skillet. Cook on both sides at medium-high heat until browned. Top with fresh fruit, yogurt, or a spoonful of maple syrup.

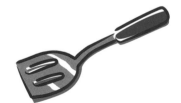

Adam's apricot-raisin oatmeal

MAKES A SINGLE SERVING

- ½ cup oatmeal or multigrain cereal
- Sprinkle of raisins
- 2 tablespoons chopped dried apricots
- ½ teaspoon cinnamon
- ¾ cup water

Mix ingredients in microwavable bowl or stove-top saucepan. Cook until soft, then cool and serve with milk. Top with a teaspoon of maple syrup. Feel free to add or substitute chopped apples, pears, blueberries, or any fruit that is in season.

Lunches for the toddler bunch

It's lunchtime already? Whether it seems like the day has flown by or it feels like you've been up for two days before the noonish hour strikes, lunch is an important part of the day for your toddler. It provides additional nutrition, routine, and a prelude to naptime. If you need some inspiration beyond chopped banana and cheese toast or are out of refrigerated leftovers, try some of the quick, easy-to-prepare, and healthy recipes below.

Five-minute pizza

MAKES A SINGLE SERVING

- 1 whole wheat English muffin half
- 1 tablespoon tomato paste or sauce
- 1 tablespoon grated carrot or other favorite veggie
- 1 slice cheese

Spread the muffin with the tomato paste or sauce. Top with the carrot and cheese. Bake at 400° F for 5 minutes until the cheese melts. Cut into small pieces and serve with chopped fruit. *(See photo on opposite page.)*

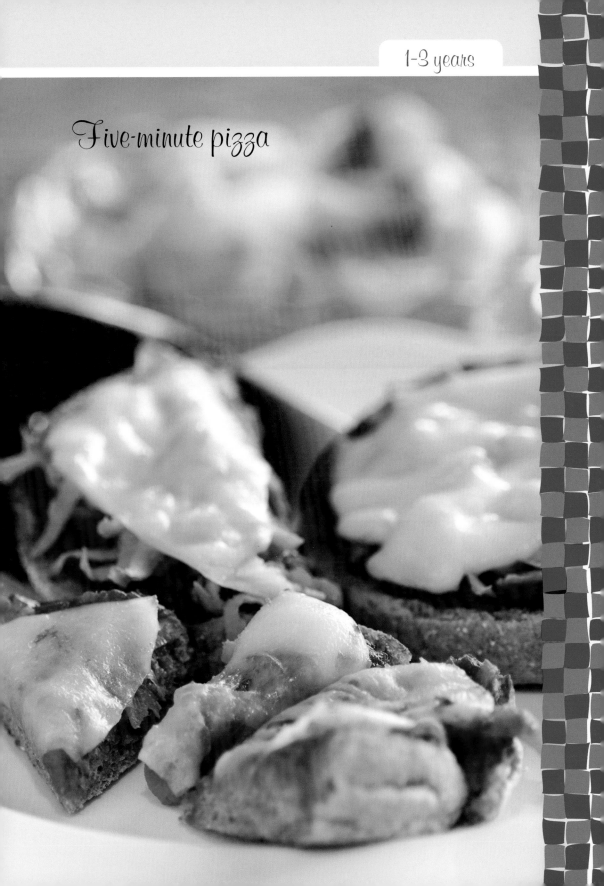

Five-minute pizza

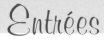

Chopped chicken salad

MAKES 3 SERVINGS

- ½ cup plain low-fat yogurt
- 2 teaspoons apple cider vinegar
- 1 teaspoon honey
- 1 cup seedless grapes, halved
- 1 celery stalk, chopped
- 1 to 2 cooked, diced chicken breasts

Remember, no honey for children less than one year old.

Mix yogurt, vinegar, and honey. Toss with the rest of the ingredients. Serve. The yogurt mixture is good alone, too. *(See photo on opposite page.)*

Pita pockets

MAKES 3 SERVINGS

- ¼ cup leftover cooked tender meat or fish, such as sole or tilapia
- 1 to 2 tablespoons plain yogurt
- 1 tablespoon chopped tomato
- Dash of salt and pepper
- 1 whole wheat pita
- 2 tablespoons grated Jack or cheddar cheese

Chop meat or flake fish and mix it with yogurt, tomato, salt, and pepper. Stuff into pita and top mixture with grated cheese. Cook pita on both sides in an oiled frying pan or bake in a 350° F oven for 10 minutes or until cheese melts. Cut into bite-sized pieces.

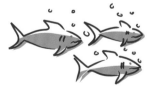

Chopped chicken salad

Open-faced cranberry turkey melt

MAKES 1-2 SERVINGS

- 1 slice whole wheat bread
- 1 tablespoon soft cream cheese
- Spinach leaves
- 1 tablespoon jellied cranberry sauce
- 2 slices fresh roasted turkey
- 1 slice provolone or mozzarella cheese

Preheat oven to 350° F. Spread bread with cream cheese. Layer with a single layer of spinach, cranberry sauce, turkey, and provolone or mozzarella. Bake 5 to 10 minutes or until cheese melts. Cut into small bites and serve. *(See photo on opposite page.)*

Optional: Add slices of avocado. Substitute 9-inch whole wheat flour tortilla for bread and prepare as a wrap.

P'ba & honeywich*

MAKES 2 SERVINGS

- 4 tablespoons 100 percent peanut butter or almond butter
- 2 teaspoons honey
- 2 slices whole-grain bread

Mix peanut butter and honey and spread thinly on one piece of bread. Cover with the second piece of bread, and cut into mini-sandwiches.

Add sliced banana if you wish.

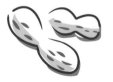

*Do not serve to children who are allergic to nuts! Remember, no honey for children less than one year old.

Open-faced cranberry turkey melt

Lemony carrot salad

MAKES 3-4 SERVINGS

- 2 large carrots, grated
- ½ cup lemon yogurt

Mix and serve! You may try substituting plain yogurt for lemon yogurt and add ¼ cup raisins as a variation. *(See photo on opposite page.)*

Molasses chicken cantaloupe salad

MAKES 3-4 SERVINGS

- 1 tablespoon blackstrap molasses
- 1 tablespoon grade B maple syrup
- 1½ tablespoons low-sodium soy sauce
- 3 tablespoons canola oil
- ¼ teaspoon cinnamon
- 1 cooked chicken breast, chopped
- ½ cup fresh or defrosted cantaloupe cubes

Whisk the first five ingredients together and toss with the chicken and cantaloupe. Serve.

This recipe is packed with protein, iron, vitamin C, and healthy fats.

Vegan version: Substitute chicken with chopped extra-firm tofu.

Adam's antipasto

MAKES 1-2 SERVINGS

- 1 chopped, cooked turkey sausage or sliced low-sodium deli turkey
- 1 sliced hard-boiled egg
- 4 cherry tomato halves
- 1 ounce mozzarella cheese, diced

Arrange on toddler plate and serve!

Lemony carrot salad

Freckled eggs

MAKES 6 SERVINGS

- 3 hard-boiled eggs
- 2 teaspoons mustard
- 2 tablespoons plain yogurt
- 1 tablespoon sweet pickle relish
- Paprika

Peel and slice the eggs in half. Remove the yolks and mash in a small bowl with all of the ingredients except for the paprika. Spoon the yolk mixture into the egg white halves. Sprinkle with paprika. *(See photo on opposite page.)*

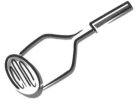

Grant-man's mash

MAKES 2–3 SERVINGS

- 1 large potato, peeled
- ½ cup broccoli florets
- ½ cup milk
- 1 tablespoon olive oil
- ¼ cup grated white cheddar cheese

Boil, microwave, or steam the potato and broccoli until soft. Purée or finely chop the broccoli. Mash the potato. Blend all ingredients.

For extra calcium, add 1 tablespoon dry milk powder.

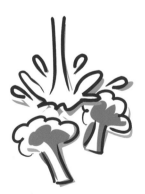

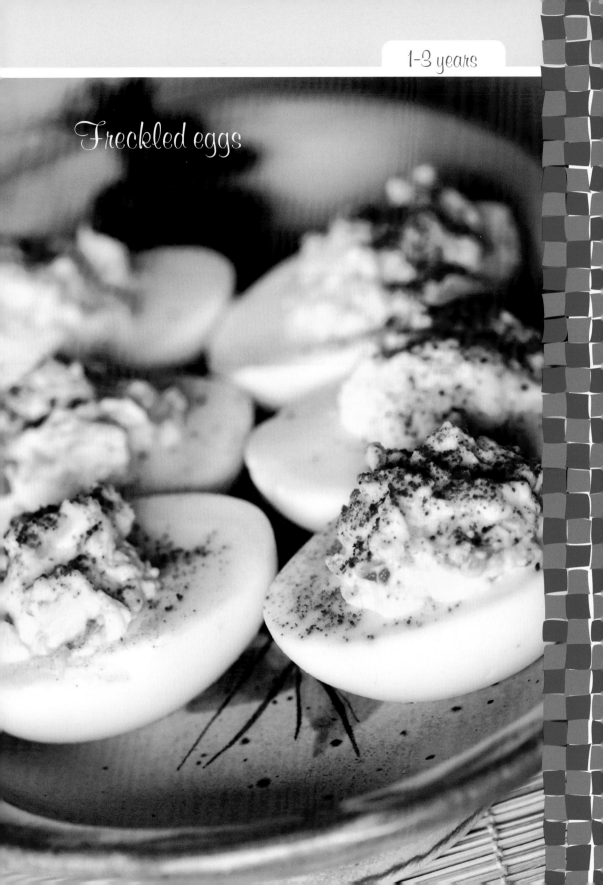

Freckled eggs

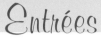

Flavor-infused noodles

Cook your favorite noodles in chicken or vegetable broth and drain until noodles are just wet. Add sliced carrots and cubed chicken or tofu for a full meal. No time? Buy a can of low-salt organic vegetable-noodle soup, heat, drain most of the broth, and serve. (See Appendix 2, Shopping Simplicity, page 149.)

Gracie's tofu
MAKES 2–3 SERVINGS

- 4 ounces extra-firm tofu
- Tamari or soy sauce

Chop the tofu and sprinkle it with soy sauce. Serve with chopped or sliced seasonal fruit.

Quesadilla corners
MAKES 2–3 SERVINGS

- ¼ cup refried beans
- 2 tablespoons finely chopped veggies (tomato, bell pepper, sweet onion, broccoli florets)
- 2 soft flour tortillas
- 3 tablespoons grated Jack or cheddar cheese

Mix the beans with the veggies. Spread onto one tortilla. Top with cheese. Cover with the other tortilla. Bake in 350° F oven for 5 to 10 minutes. Cut into small triangles.

Dinner: Day's end toddler edibles

Dinner is an important meal for toddlers, not only to expose them to more nutritious foods but to provide the opportunity to sit down together as a family. Even if your toddlers typically only eat about a quarter of the food on their plate, they still benefit from this time to interact and feel a part of the family dinner dynamic. All Toddler Bistro meals include the Chef's choice of meat, fish, or vegan protein and a vegetable, followed by a complimentary Sippycuppo'latte (sippy cup of milk).

Chickpea–sweet potato cakes   MAKES APPROXIMATELY 10 CAKES

- 1 large sweet potato or yam
- 1 cup cooked chickpeas (garbanzo beans)
- 2 tablespoons tamari or soy sauce
- 1 teaspoon olive oil
- ½ teaspoon cumin
- 1 teaspoon grated fresh ginger
- 1 teaspoon pepper
- 1 tablespoon all-purpose flour
- 1 cup cooked brown rice
- 1 medium carrot, grated
- 1 small zucchini, grated

Poke holes in the sweet potato or yam with a fork. Bake, wrapped in foil, at 425° F for 60 minutes, or microwave on a root vegetable setting—about 5 to 6 minutes on high. Test with a fork to make sure that the flesh is cooked through and soft. Peel and mash it in a large bowl with the chickpeas. Add the rest of the ingredients and mix well. Form into small patties. Place on an oiled baking sheet and bake at 350° F for 15 minutes on each side.

71

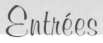

All veggie spaghetti

MAKES 8 SERVINGS

- 1- to 2-pound spaghetti squash
- 2 cups organic garden vegetable tomato sauce or your favorite spaghetti sauce
- 3 tablespoons grated Parmesan cheese

Preheat the oven to 350° F. Cut squash in half, remove seeds, and place cut side down on a baking sheet. Bake until tender, about 45 minutes. Turn once during cooking. For microwave cooking, place squash cut side down in a glass dish with ¼ cup water. Cover with microwave plastic wrap and cook 7–10 minutes. With a fork, scrape the strands of squash from each half into a large serving bowl. Toss with tomato sauce and top with Parmesan cheese. *(See photo on opposite page.)*

Variations: Toss with 1 tablespoon butter and 4 tablespoons Parmesan cheese. Add in cooked peas and chopped, cooked carrots. For a meat version, add cooked ground meat or diced chicken breast.

Golden roasted veggies

MAKES 6 SERVINGS

- 1 sweet potato or yam, sliced into ½-inch-thick rounds
- 1 medium winter squash (acorn, butternut), sliced into ¼-inch rings and seeded
- 1 bunch baby carrots
- ¼ cup olive oil
- Dash of salt and pepper

Toss the veggies in the olive oil. Sprinkle with salt and pepper. Place in a single layer on a large oiled baking sheet with sides. Bake at 400° F for 30 to 35 minutes until golden brown and tender. Turn the veggies after 15 minutes to ensure even browning.

Cook as many or as few veggies as you want. Serve like French fries with a little ketchup or with grated cheese. Save extras for snacks.

All veggie spaghetti

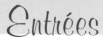

The unfishy fish sticks

MAKES 4–6 SERVINGS

- 1 egg
- ¼ cup ketchup
- 1 tablespoon soy sauce
- 2 to 3 firm white fish fillets (cod, halibut, or flounder)
- ½ cup all-purpose flour
- 1 cup dried whole wheat bread crumbs

Preheat the oven to 425° F. Mix the egg, ketchup, and soy sauce together. Cut the fish fillets into 1-inch pieces. Dust with flour. Dip in the egg mixture. Roll in the bread crumbs. Bake on an oiled baking sheet for 10 minutes.

You may substitute chicken strips, turkey, or firm tofu slices for fish. If you choose a more tender fish such as sole or tilapia, follow the recipe but do not cut the fish into strips until it is baked.

Speedy spinach frittata

MAKES 12 SERVINGS

- ¼ cup dried whole wheat bread crumbs
- 1 cup grated cheddar cheese
- 1 10-ounce package frozen chopped spinach, thawed and drained
- 1 cup cottage cheese
- 3 eggs, beaten
- 1 tablespoon olive oil
- 1 teaspoon nutmeg
- ¼ cup grated Parmesan cheese
- Dash of salt and pepper

Set aside 2 tablespoons of the bread crumbs and ¼ cup of the cheddar cheese. Mix the rest of the ingredients in a large bowl. Sprinkle the bottom of a square oiled baking dish with the reserved bread crumbs. Spread on the spinach mixture. Sprinkle with the reserved cheese and bake at 350° F for 45 minutes. *(See photo on opposite page.)*

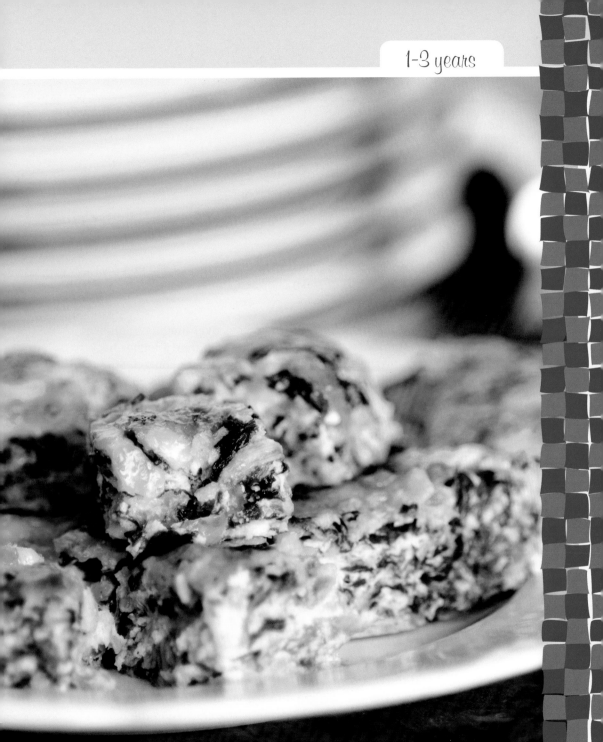

Speedy spinach frittata

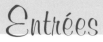

Power packin' purée

MAKES 16 SERVINGS

- 1 28-ounce can whole tomatoes
- 2 cans chickpeas (garbanzo beans)
- 2 teaspoons minced garlic
- 1 teaspoon ginger
- 1 teaspoon cumin
- Dash of salt and pepper
- 1 10-ounce package frozen chopped spinach, thawed and drained, or 2 pounds of fresh chopped spinach
- 1 tablespoon lemon juice

Simmer the tomatoes, beans, garlic, and spices over medium-high heat for 10 minutes. Transfer to a food processor and purée. Transfer back to the pot and stir in the spinach and lemon juice until cooked. Spread on bread or pita pieces, or serve as a soup. Top with grated cheese.

Cheesy chicken fingers

MAKES 8 SERVINGS

- ¼ cup olive oil
- 1 cup fine, dried whole wheat bread crumbs
- ½ cup grated mozzarella cheese
- 1 teaspoon minced garlic
- 1 tablespoon paprika
- ½ cup plain yogurt
- 1 tablespoon Worcestershire sauce
- 1 teaspoon celery salt
- 4 boneless chicken breasts, cut into 1-inch strips

Pour the olive oil into a baking dish. Mix the bread crumbs and cheese in one bowl and the rest of the ingredients (except for the chicken) in a separate bowl. Dip the chicken into the yogurt mixture, then roll in the bread crumb/cheese mixture. Arrange the chicken in the baking dish and bake at 450° F for 20 minutes.

You may substitute turkey cutlets for chicken.

Tortellini and trees

MAKES 4–5 SERVINGS

- 1 package cheese or chicken and cheese tortellini (look for spinach or tricolor pasta)
- 1 10-ounce package frozen organic broccoli
- 2 teaspoons extra-virgin olive oil
- ½ cup grated Parmesan cheese

Cook tortellini as directed. Place the frozen broccoli in your sieve for draining the pasta. When the pasta is done, pour it over the broccoli in the sieve. As the water drains through, it will defrost and heat the broccoli. Transfer the pasta and broccoli to a bowl and toss with olive oil and cheese. Serve!

Sweet potato patties

MAKES APPROXIMATELY 8 PATTIES

- 1 large sweet potato
- 1 tablespoon milk
- 1 egg, beaten
- 1 tablespoon olive oil
- 2 tablespoons all-purpose flour
- ½ cup sweet onion, minced
- ½ cup zucchini, grated
- 1 teaspoon fresh ginger, grated
- Dash of salt and pepper
- Vegetable oil spray
- 1 to 2 cups dried whole wheat bread crumbs

Poke holes in the sweet potato with a fork. Bake it, wrapped in foil, at 425° F for 60 minutes, or microwave it on a root vegetable setting—about 5 to 6 minutes on high. Test with a fork to make sure that the flesh is cooked through and soft. Lower oven temperature or preheat to 350° F. Scoop out the inside and mash with all of the ingredients except for the bread crumbs. Form into small balls, roll in the bread crumbs, and pat flat on a lightly oiled baking sheet. Bake for 15 minutes on each side.

You may substitute yams for sweet potatoes.

Adam's "cupcake" salmon puffs

MAKES 6 SERVINGS

- 1 egg
- ½ cup milk
- 2 cups canned salmon
- 1 tablespoon lemon juice
- ½ cup dried whole wheat bread crumbs
- 1 tablespoon olive oil
- 2 tablespoons grated sweet onion
- 1 teaspoon pepper
- ¼ teaspoon salt

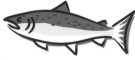

Beat the egg and milk in a medium bowl. Mix in the rest of the ingredients. Spoon into an oiled 6-muffin baking tin. Bake at 350° F for 30 to 35 minutes. Serve with a favorite dip. (Pink Dip is great! See Dips, Sauces, and Spreads Galore, page 105.) *(See photo on opposite page.)*

The meatless meatloaf

MAKES 6–8 SERVINGS

- 1½ cups textured vegetable protein
- 2 cups boiling water
- 6 scallions, sliced, green tops removed
- 1 carrot, grated
- 1 cup dried whole wheat bread crumbs or
  1 cup cooked brown rice
- 2 teaspoons sesame oil
- 1 teaspoon minced garlic
- 2 tablespoons grated fresh ginger
- 2 tablespoons tamari or soy sauce
- Optional: Add 1 grated small zucchini or yellow squash

Combine the first two ingredients and stir until the water is absorbed. Mix with the rest of the ingredients. Place in an oiled loaf pan. Bake at 375° F for 20 minutes. For a nonvegetarian version, substitute 1¼ pounds of lean ground meat for textured vegetable protein and water and increase the baking time to 45 minutes.

Adam's "cupcake" salmon puffs

Toddler tempting turkey meatloaf

MAKES 6–8 SERVINGS

- 1¼ pounds lean ground turkey
- 1 large carrot, grated
- ¼ cup finely chopped sweet onions
- 1 10-ounce package frozen chopped spinach, thawed and drained
- 2 slices whole wheat bread, torn into small pieces
- 1 egg, lightly beaten
- 1 teaspoon Worcestershire sauce
- ½ teaspoon minced garlic
- ½ teaspoon nutmeg
- Dash of salt and pepper
- 3 tablespoons grated Parmesan cheese
- 1 teaspoon grated lemon rind

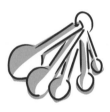

Preheat the oven to 350˚ F. Mix all of the ingredients in a bowl, form into a loaf, and place in an oiled loaf pan. Bake for 45 to 50 minutes. Yummy! *(See photo on opposite page.)*

You may substitute lean ground beef for turkey, or vegans may substitute 1½ cups of textured vegetable protein soaked in 2 cups of boiling water.

Roasted squash stars

MAKES 4 SERVINGS

- 1 acorn squash
- 2 tablespoons olive oil
- Dash of salt and pepper

Slice the squash horizontally into 1-inch-wide pieces. Remove the seeds. Toss the slices in olive oil and bake them on a foil-covered baking sheet at 400˚ F for 20 minutes or until soft. Sprinkle with salt and pepper.

Sweet version: Substitute a little brown sugar and cinnamon for the salt and pepper.

Toddler tempting turkey meatloaf

Cheesy zucchini muffins

MAKES TWO DOZEN MUFFINS

- 2 cups all-purpose flour
- 1 cup whole wheat flour
- 4 teaspoons baking powder
- ½ teaspoon baking soda
- 1 teaspoon salt
- 2 eggs
- 1 cup low-fat buttermilk
- ¼ cup canola oil
- 3 tablespoons chopped parsley
- 1 cup grated zucchini
- 1 cup grated cheddar cheese

Sift the dry ingredients into a large bowl. Beat the eggs with milk and oil and combine with the rest of the ingredients. Mix into the dry ingredients. Spoon the mixture into lined or oiled regular-sized muffin tins until they are three-quarters full. Bake at 350° F for 30 minutes.

To make bread instead of muffins, use a 9-inch-square oiled baking dish. Bake for 35 to 40 minutes. Poke the center with a toothpick to see if the bread is baked through. The toothpick should come out clean if it is. Cut the bread into squares and serve.

Parsnip mashed potatoes

MAKES 2–3 SERVINGS

- 1 large russet potato, peeled
- 1 parsnip
- 1 cup milk
- ¼ teaspoon salt
- 1 tablespoon olive oil

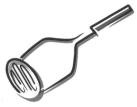

Cut the potato and parsnip into chunks. Place in a pot or microwavable dish and add water or broth to cover. Cook until soft, mash, and blend in the rest of the ingredients. Great for those in the white-food funk!

Asian-fusion flapjacks

MAKES 4 SERVINGS

- 1 red bell pepper
- 1 small sweet onion or 3 scallions (green tops removed)
- ½ cup water chestnuts
- 2 medium carrots
- 1 zucchini
- 3 eggs, lightly beaten
- ¼ teaspoon salt
- 1 tablespoon baking powder
- ½ cup whole wheat flour
- 1 tablespoon tamari or soy sauce
- Vegetable oil spray

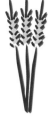

Chop the bell pepper, onion, and water chestnuts by hand or with a food processor. Grate the carrot and zucchini. Mix all of the ingredients in a large bowl. Form into patties using ¼ cup of mixture for each patty. Cook on both sides in an oiled skillet until nicely browned. Serve with your favorite sauce (see Dips, Sauces, and Spreads Galore, page 105).

Tasty toddler grilled tofu

MAKES 4-6 SERVINGS

- 8 to 14 ounces extra-firm tofu
- 2 tablespoons lemon juice
- 1 teaspoon grated fresh ginger
- 2 tablespoons tamari or soy sauce
- 2 tablespoons orange juice
- ½ teaspoon curry powder
- 2 teaspoons minced garlic
- 2 tablespoons ketchup
- 1½ tablespoons molasses

Slice the tofu into 1-inch pieces. Mix the rest of the ingredients and marinate for 2 or more hours in the fridge. Place on a lightly oiled baking pan. Bake 12 minutes on each side in a 400° F oven or until golden brown. You may substitute chicken or fish for the tofu.

Quick broccoli and cheese no-crust quiche

MAKES 8 SERVINGS

- 1 10-ounce package frozen broccoli florets
- 6 large eggs
- ½ cup milk
- 1 teaspoon nutmeg
- ¼ teaspoon pepper
- ½ teaspoon salt
- 1 cup grated cheddar cheese

Cook the broccoli for 1 minute in boiling water or microwave it. Drain and chop. Whisk together the eggs, milk, and spices. Stir in the broccoli and cheese. Coat a 9-inch pie dish with vegetable oil spray. Pour in the mixture. Bake at 350° F for 35 to 40 minutes. *(See photo on opposite page.)*

Primo pasta primavera

MAKES 4 SERVINGS

- ½ pound whole wheat penne or shell pasta
- 2 tablespoons olive oil
- 1 teaspoon minced garlic
- 1 small red bell pepper, cut into bite-sized strips
- ¼ cup sliced mushrooms
- ½ cup broccoli florets
- 1 tablespoon lemon juice

Cook the pasta. Heat the oil and garlic in a pan and sauté the veggies over medium heat. Stir in the lemon juice. Toss the veggies with the pasta.

Option: Toss with marinara, grated Parmesan or other favorite cheeses, or Cheesy Sauce from Dips, Sauces, and Spreads Galore, page 105. To save time, substitute a 10-ounce bag of frozen organic chopped veggies for the sautéed veggies. Pour the veggies into the bottom of the sieve that you use for draining the cooked pasta. The hot pasta water will defrost and warm the veggies as it passes through the sieve.

Quick broccoli and
cheese no-crust quiche

Mouth-watering Midwest BBQ

MAKES 5 SERVINGS

- 2 tablespoons water
- ½ teaspoon mustard
- 1 teaspoon Worcestershire sauce
- 1 tablespoon honey
- 2 tablespoons apple cider vinegar
- 1 teaspoon chili pepper
- 2 to 3 chicken breasts, cooked and shredded

In a medium saucepan, combine all of the ingredients except for the chicken. Stir on medium-low heat until simmering. Add the shredded chicken and heat through, stirring in extra water if necessary. Serve with Parsnip Mashed Potatoes or Golden Roasted Veggies (see pages 82 and 72). Keep leftovers for quesadillas or pizzas.

Remember, no honey for children less than one year old.

Spinach-pesto chicken pizza

MAKES 16 SERVINGS

- 1 10-ounce package frozen chopped spinach, thawed and squeezed dry
- 1 egg white
- 8 ounces ricotta cheese
- 1 teaspoon minced garlic
- ½ cup chopped tomato
- 1 teaspoon nutmeg
- Dash of salt and pepper
- 2 to 3 cooked, chopped chicken breasts
- Premade whole wheat pizza dough for 1 pizza
- ¼ cup favorite grated cheese
- 3 tablespoons grated Parmesan cheese

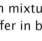

Mix all of the ingredients except for the chicken, dough, and grated cheese. Roll out the dough on a lightly oiled pizza pan. Sprinkle the chicken over the dough and top with the spinach mixture, then the grated cheese. Bake at 400° F for 20 minutes. Offer in bite-sized pieces.

Delicious dippin' chicken

MAKES 6 SERVINGS

- 2 eggs, beaten
- 1 cup frozen chopped spinach, thawed and squeezed dry
- ¾ cup grated Parmesan cheese
- 1 teaspoon minced garlic
- ¼ teaspoon pepper
- 2 teaspoons Italian herbs
- ½ teaspoon salt
- 3 to 4 chicken breasts
- ½ cup all-purpose flour

Mix all of the ingredients together except for the chicken and flour. Dip the chicken breasts in the flour and dust off the excess. Dip in the batter and bake in an oiled dish for 20 to 30 minutes at 450° F. Slice the breasts into 1-inch pieces and serve plain or with your toddler's favorite dipping sauce from Dips, Sauces, and Spreads Galore, page 105.

Savory spinach tofu saag

MAKES 4-6 SERVINGS

- 1 medium sweet onion
- 2 tablespoons olive oil
- 1 teaspoon ground ginger
- 2 teaspoons coriander seed
- ½ teaspoon turmeric
- 1 cinnamon stick
- 1 pound fresh spinach
- 1 cup water
- 1 teaspoon lemon juice
- ½ teaspoon salt
- 1 cup plain full-fat yogurt
- 1 8-ounce package of regular tofu, chopped

Sauté onion in oil until it becomes translucent. Add the spices and sauté for another 2 to 3 minutes. Add a little water if necessary. Add the spinach, 1 cup of water, the lemon juice, and the salt, and simmer for

10 to 15 minutes over low heat. Remove from heat and allow to cool a bit. Then use a blender or food processor to purée (remove the cinnamon stick). Return the purée to the pot. Replace the cinnamon stick. Add more water if necessary. Simmer another 5 to 10 minutes. Stir in the yogurt and tofu and return to briefly simmer. Do not boil. Add extra seasoning for adult servings.

Family falafel
MAKES 4 SERVINGS

- ¼ cup thinly sliced scallion with green tops removed
- 2 teaspoons minced garlic
- 1 tablespoon olive oil
- ½ pound lean ground beef or turkey
- ¼ teaspoon balsamic vinegar
- 1 cup chopped celery
- 1 large tomato, chopped
- ¼ cup raisins
- ¾ teaspoon sugar
- ¾ teaspoon oregano
- ½ teaspoon cumin
- 1 teaspoon salt
- Dash of pepper

Sauté the onion and garlic in oil. Add the meat, brown, and drain the fat if there is any. Stir in the rest of the ingredients, cover, and simmer for 20 to 25 minutes. Serve with whole wheat pita bread, in a cheese quesadilla, or plain with a favorite sauce. *(See photo on opposite page.)*

For extra nutrients, add sliced mushrooms or a chopped apple.

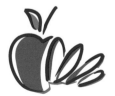

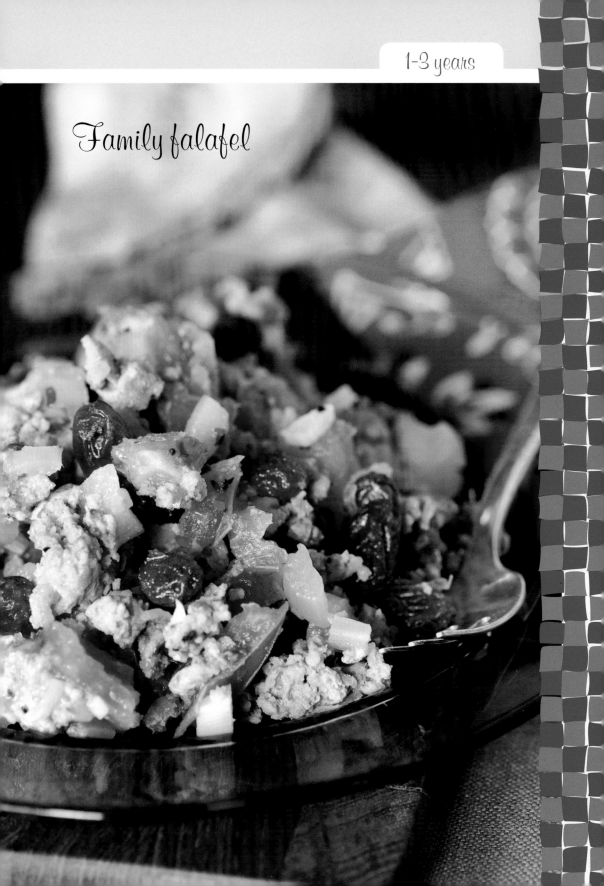

Family falafel

Summer vegetable picnic pizza

MAKES 12–16 SERVINGS

Topping:
- 2 tablespoons olive oil
- 1 sweet yellow onion, chopped
- 1 12-ounce can chopped organic tomatoes, drained
- 1 teaspoon tomato paste
- 1 tablespoon fresh, minced thyme or 1 teaspoon dried thyme

- Dash of pepper
- 1 red bell pepper and 1 yellow bell pepper, seeded and chopped
- 1 zucchini, thinly sliced (Hint: Use the side of a cheese grater)
- 5½ cups baby spinach leaves
- 1 cup chopped, cooked chicken breast or extra-firm tofu
- 1 cup grated mozzarella cheese

Crust:
- 1¾ cups whole wheat flour
- 1¾ cups unbleached, all-purpose flour plus extra for dusting
- 1 teaspoon brown sugar
- 1 teaspoon baking soda
- 1 teaspoon sea salt
- 1½ cups buttermilk

Heat 1 tablespoon of oil in a large skillet and sauté the onion until soft. Add the tomatoes, tomato paste, thyme, and pepper. Simmer down to a thick sauce, which will take approximately 30 minutes. Remove from heat and cool. Heat the last tablespoon of oil in the skillet and cook the bell peppers and zucchini until just brown. Cool. Put the spinach in a colander and pour boiling water over the leaves to wilt. Squeeze dry and mince.

Preheat the oven to 425° F. Mix the flours, sugar, baking soda, and salt in a large bowl, and add the buttermilk. Once you have formed the dough, turn it out onto a floured board and knead briefly. Divide the dough into 6 pieces. Roll out each piece into a 5-inch circle and place on oiled baking sheets. Spread with the tomato sauce and top with the spinach, bell peppers, zucchini, chicken, and cheese. Bake in a preheated oven for 25 minutes.

Remove from the oven and serve, refrigerate, or freeze for summer picnics. Enjoy!

Time-saving tip: Skip the sauce and dough preparation and use low-salt, premade pizza sauce and premade whole wheat pizza dough. Top the pizza with the remaining ingredients.

Ricotta rice quiche

MAKES 8 SERVINGS

- 2 tablespoons olive oil
- ½ sweet onion, chopped
- 1 zucchini, grated, or a 10-ounce bag frozen, chopped mixed veggies, thawed
- ½ cup chopped red bell pepper
- 1 cup chopped broccoli or cauliflower
- 1 cup cooked brown or converted rice
- 1 teaspoon dried basil
- ½ teaspoon salt
- 1 cup ricotta cheese
- 2 eggs
- 1 cup grated Jack cheese
- 1 tablespoon wheat germ

Heat the oil and cook the onion and veggies for about 5 minutes or until tender. Stir in rice and spices. Beat the ricotta, eggs, and half of the Jack cheese in a separate bowl. Oil a 9-inch pie dish. Sprinkle the wheat germ on the bottom. Spoon in half of the rice mixture. Spread the ricotta mixture on top. Top with the rest of the rice mixture, then the rest of the cheese. Bake at 350° F for 30 to 35 minutes.

Wholesome chicken squares

MAKES 8 SQUARES

- 2 tablespoons light whipped cream cheese
- 2 tablespoons melted butter or margarine (trans fat-free)
- 1 12.5-ounce can low-sodium white-chunk chicken
- 2 tablespoons minced sweet onion
- ½ cup chopped celery
- ½ teaspoon salt
- 1 teaspoon pepper
- 1 tablespoon chopped parsley
  (Optional: Add more for some extra green!)
- 1 package whole wheat pizza dough

Preheat the oven to 450° F. Blend the cream cheese and butter or margarine in a medium-sized bowl. Mix in the rest of the ingredients, except for the dough. Roll out the dough, into a ¼-inch-thick layer on a floured cutting board. Cut the dough into square shapes, approximately 4 inch squares. Spoon ½-cup portions of the chicken mixture onto each square and pull the opposite corners of the dough over the chicken, pinching the ends together. Bake on an oiled cookie sheet for 15 minutes or until golden. Cool. Cut into bite-sized pieces and serve!

This recipe is a healthier revamp of my childhood favorite. Leftovers are great for lunches! *(See photo on opposite page.)*

Perfect patty melt

MAKES 1–2 SERVINGS

- 1 tablespoon tomato paste or sauce
- 1 whole-grain English muffin half
- 1 soy-based sausage patty or 1 slice regular cooked meat
- 2 slices avocado
- 1 slice of soy or regular cheese

Spread the sauce on the muffin half and top with the meat and avocado, then the cheese. Bake in a 350° F oven until the cheese melts. Cool, cut into bite-sized pieces, and serve.

Wholesome
chicken squares

Creamy sweet potato–pumpkin soup

MAKES 10 SERVINGS

- 1 tablespoon olive oil
- 1 cup chopped yellow onion
- 1 teaspoon ginger
- ½ teaspoon curry powder
- ¼ teaspoon cumin
- ¼ teaspoon nutmeg
- 2 garlic cloves, minced
- 2 cups peeled, cubed sweet potato
- 2 cups low-sodium chicken broth
- 1½ cups water
- 1 15-ounce can pureéd pumpkin*
- 1 cup milk
- 5 tablespoons plain yogurt

Heat the olive oil in a large pot over medium-high heat. Add the onion and sauté until translucent and tender. Stir in the spices and garlic and cook for 1 to 2 minutes. Add the sweet potato, broth, water, and pumpkin. Bring to a boil. Reduce heat and simmer for 20 minutes or until the sweet potato is soft. Remove from heat and stir in the milk. Transfer to a food processor and purée. Serve topped with ½ table-spoon of plain yogurt per serving.

Make a face or swirl yogurt in a fun design for toddlers to enjoy!

Vegans may substitute soy milk, soy yogurt, and veggie broth.

* Try to choose organic brands if possible.

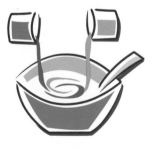

Snacks: The Toddler Bistro lighter fare

Snacks are an important part of toddlers' diets, and for some children, they make up the bulk of their daily nutrition. Some of these recipes are great for quick single servings, while others make a big batch that can be munched on for the week or frozen for later.

Cinnamony yogurt

MAKES A SINGLE SERVING

- ¼ cup plain yogurt
- 1 teaspoon cinnamon
- ½ teaspoon honey
- ¼ teaspoon vanilla

Mix and serve!

Remember, no honey for children less than one year old.

Cinnamon-maple butternut browns

MAKES 8–10 SERVINGS

- 2½ cups butternut squash, cut into 1-inch cubes
- 2 tablespoons canola oil
- 1 tablespoon maple syrup
- ½ teaspoon ground cinnamon
- ½ cup dried whole wheat bread crumbs

Preheat the oven to 425° F. In a 13 x 9-inch baking dish, toss the squash with oil, syrup, and cinnamon. Lightly toss in the bread crumbs. Spread the squash evenly into a single layer in the dish. Bake for 10 minutes on each side.

Tip: Trader Joe's, Whole Foods, and other health markets carry precut butternut squash cubes.

Awesome avocado bread

MAKES 8–10 SERVINGS

- 2 eggs, beaten
- 1 cup mashed avocados
- ½ cup canola oil
- ¾ cup sugar
- 2 teaspoons lemon juice
- ½ teaspoon salt
- 2 teaspoon baking powder
- 1 cup all purpose flour
- ½ cup whole wheat flour
- ½ teaspoon cinnamon
- ½ teaspoon cloves
- ½ cup chopped walnuts*

*Omit walnuts for children who are allergic to nuts.

Mix the eggs with the avocado. Add the oil and sugar, then the rest of the ingredients. Pour into a 9 x 5-inch oiled and floured loaf pan. Bake at 350˚F for 15 minutes, then at 325˚F for 45 minutes, or until a toothpick inserted into the bread comes out clean.

Grant's great pumpkin custard

MAKES 8 SERVINGS

- 1 16-ounce can puréed pumpkin*
- 1 egg plus 2 egg whites
- 1 12-ounce can evaporated milk
  (use nonfat for two- to three-year-olds)
- ¾ cup maple syrup
- ½ teaspoon nutmeg
- ½ teaspoon ginger
- 1 teaspoon cinnamon

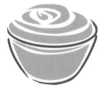

Blend all of the ingredients. Pour into an oiled 1-quart baking dish. Bake at 350˚F for 45 to 60 minutes until an inserted knife comes out clean.

* Try to choose organic brands if possible.

Pronto apple-pumpkin bars

MAKES ABOUT TWO DOZEN BARS

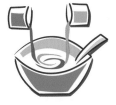

- ¾ cup packed brown sugar
- 1 rounded cup whole wheat flour
- 1 cup all-purpose flour
- 2 teaspoons cinnamon
- 2 teaspoons baking powder
- 1 teaspoon baking soda
- ½ teaspoon salt
- ½ cup applesauce
- ½ cup canola oil
- 1 16-ounce can puréed pumpkin
- 3 eggs
- 1 teaspoon vanilla

Mix the dry ingredients. Stir in the wet ingredients. Pour into an oiled 15 x 10 x 1-inch jelly roll pan or large rectangular baking dish. Bake at 350° F for 30 minutes.

Cut into favorite shapes!

Baked veggie crisps

MAKES 8-10 SERVINGS

- 1 small potato
- 1 small sweet potato
- 1 parsnip
- 1 carrot
- 2 tablespoons olive oil
- Dash of salt and pepper

Thinly slice the veggies. Toss in the olive oil. Place on an oiled baking sheet and sprinkle with salt and pepper. Bake at 400° F for 10 minutes or until crisp. Toss halfway through baking.

Best baked apples

MAKES 2 SERVINGS

- 1 or more large firm apples, Fuji or other baking variety
- 1 teaspoon butter
- 1 teaspoon cinnamon
- 1 tablespoon maple syrup

Wash and core the apples. Mix and add the rest of the ingredients into the apples' hollow centers. Place upright in a glass baking dish with about ¼ inch of water to prevent burning. Microwave in a covered dish or bake at 425° F until soft (approximately 45 minutes). *(See photo on opposite page.)*

Yummy hummus

MAKES APPROXIMATELY 12 SERVINGS

- 1 can chickpeas (garbanzo beans), drained
- 2 teaspoons lemon juice
- 1 teaspoon minced garlic
- ½ teaspoon salt
- 1 teaspoon curry powder
- ¼ teaspoon cumin
- 1 teaspoon pepper
- 1 tablespoon water
- 1½ teaspoons honey
- 1 tablespoon olive oil
- 1 handful fresh spinach leaves

Remember, no honey for children less than one year old.

Blend all of the ingredients in a food processor, adding the spinach last. For a thinner consistency, add more olive oil. Spread in sandwiches, on pita pieces, or on crackers.

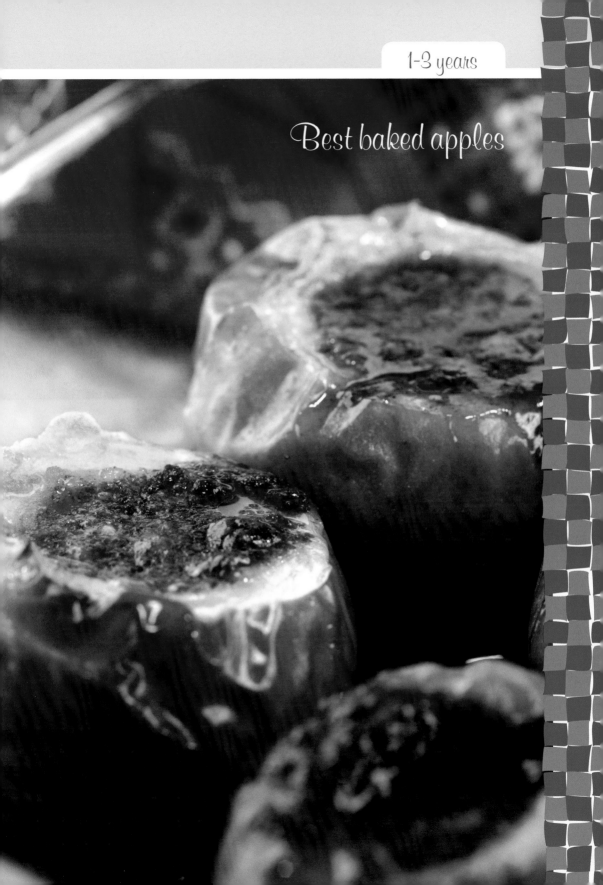

Best baked apples

Fruity yogurt smoothie

MAKES 1-2 SERVINGS

- 1 small banana
- 4 strawberries
- 1 orange
- ½ cup plain whole-fat yogurt

Combine ingredients in a blender until smooth. Pour and serve. You may also freeze the smoothie into popsicles for older children to enjoy for a healthy snack. *(See photo on opposite page.)*

Blueberry yogurt

MAKES 2-3 SERVINGS

- 1 cup plain yogurt
- ¼ cup blueberries, fresh or frozen and thawed

Blend and serve! Substitute other fruits such as diced mangoes, peaches, bananas, or strawberries.

Avocado Peach Summer Smoothie

MAKES 16 OUNCES

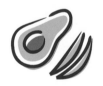

- 1 organic avocado
- 1½ cups frozen organic peaches
- ½ cup ice
- 2 tablespoons water
- 2 teaspoons fresh lemon juice
- 1 teaspoon honey

Peel avocado. Combine all ingredients in blender and mix until smooth.

Remember, no honey for children less than one year old.

Fruity yogurt smoothie

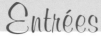

Banana-oat-apricot muffins

MAKES 4 DOZEN MINI–MUFFINS OR 12 REGULAR–SIZED MUFFINS

- 2 ripe bananas, mashed (1 cup)
- 1 egg
- 3 tablespoons canola oil
- ¾ cup plain yogurt
- 1 teaspoon vanilla
- 1 cup apple-apricot sauce or 2 4-ounce jars of apple-apricot baby food purée
- 2 cups whole wheat flour
- 1 cup brown sugar
- ¾ cup baby rolled oats
- 1 teaspoon baking soda
- 1 teaspoon baking powder
- 1 teaspoon ground nutmeg
- ½ cup chopped dried or fresh fruit (optional)

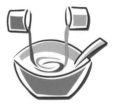

Preheat the oven to 375°F. Combine the wet ingredients in a bowl. Mix the dry ingredients in a medium-sized bowl. Stir in the wet ingredients and optional chopped fruits. Spoon the batter into oiled or lined muffin tins. Bake for 10 minutes for mini-muffins or 20 minutes for regular-sized muffins.

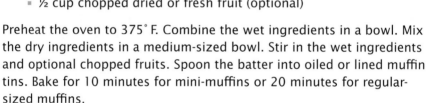

Molasses milk

MAKES A SINGLE SERVING

- 1 cup milk
- 2 teaspoons molasses

Mix and serve. Milk strikers like this one!

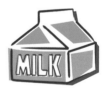

Applesauce-zucchini bran bread

MAKES 8-10 SERVINGS

- ¾ cup buttermilk
- 1 cup unsweetened applesauce
- 1 egg
- 1 cup canola oil
- 1 teaspoon vanilla
- 1 tablespoon maple syrup
- 1 cup whole wheat flour
- 1 cup all-purpose flour
- 1½ teaspoons baking soda
- ½ teaspoon baking powder
- ¼ teaspoon salt
- 1½ teaspoons cinnamon
- ½ teaspoon ginger
- ½ teaspoon nutmeg
- 1 cup packed brown sugar
- 2 cups grated zucchini*
- 1 cup bran flakes

Preheat the oven to 350° F. Combine the wet ingredients in a medium-sized bowl. Mix the dry ingredients in a small-sized bowl. Add the zucchini and bran flakes to the wet ingredients and stir in the dry ingredients. Spoon the batter into an oiled 9 x 5-inch bread pan. Bake 1 hour or until a toothpick inserted into the bread comes out clean. Cool, slice, and serve.

* Optional: Substitute 1 cup grated carrots for 1 cup grated zucchini.

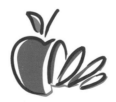

Carrot-zucchini cupcakes with citrus glaze

MAKES ONE DOZEN MUFFINS

Cupcakes:

- 1 cup whole wheat flour
- ¼ cup all-purpose flour
- 1½ teaspoons baking powder
- 1 teaspoon baking soda
- ¼ teaspoon salt
- ½ cup packed brown sugar
- 1 teaspoon cinnamon
- ¼ teaspoon nutmeg
- 1 cup grated carrot
- 1 cup grated zucchini
- 1 teaspoon grated orange rind
- 1 cup plain yogurt
- 2 eggs
- ¼ cup canola oil
- 2 tablespoons milk
- 1 teaspoon vanilla

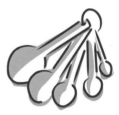

Citrus glaze:

- ½ cup sifted powdered sugar
- 1½ tablespoons fresh unsweetened orange juice
- ¼ teaspoon grated orange rind

Preheat the oven to 350° F. Mix the dry ingredients in a medium bowl. Stir in the grated carrot, zucchini, and orange rind. Mix the wet ingredients in a small bowl. Add to the flour mixture, stirring until the dry ingredients are just moistened. Spoon the batter into oiled or lined muffin tins, filling to three-quarters full. Bake for 20 minutes. Remove the cupcakes from the pan and let cool. Mix the citrus glaze ingredients together and spoon evenly over the cupcakes.

Dips, sauces, and spreads galore

Many toddlers love to dip finger foods into anything from ketchup to fondue. This can work to your advantage if you want them to eat something from which they typically turn away. My toddler nephew helped me mix three different dips and then wolfed down his salmon puff, tasting bites with each dip. It can be a little messy, but fun!

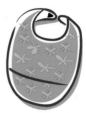

Breakfast toppers

Aside from the phenomenally strange few who don't like sweets, we tend to prefer a touch of something sweet-tasting on toast, pancakes, or cereals. Rather than train your toddler to reach for whipped butter and a bottle of artificial syrup, however, try incorporating the following naturally sweetened condiments into your breakfast menu.

- Unsweetened applesauce
- Pumpkin butter
- Apple butter
- 100 percent fruit spreads or other fruit sauce
- 1 tablespoon maple syrup
- 1 tablespoon blackstrap molasses

Yummy dips, marinades, and sauces

Here are some popular, quick dips to make from scratch. Your toddler can help you stir together ingredients for some kitchen cooking fun. You can also find some healthy, ready-made brands as well—just read the label to avoid brands high in salt (sodium) and sugars.

Pink Dip

- ¼ cup plain yogurt
- 1 tablespoon ketchup

This is a versatile dip for veggies, meatloaf, and chicken strips, or a spread for sandwiches, or to mix into canned fish or chicken. We loved tasting our salmon puffs with some pink dip, too!

Sweet ginger sauce/marinade

- 2 tablespoons tamari or soy sauce
- 2 tablespoons orange juice
- ½ teaspoon curry powder
- 1 teaspoon ginger
- 2 teaspoons minced garlic
- 2 tablespoons ketchup
- 1½ tablespoons molasses
- 2 tablespoons lemon juice

Stir together. A great marinade or sauce for chicken or tofu.

Avocado whip dip

- 1 ripe avocado, peeled and pitted
- ½ cup plain yogurt
- 1 tablespoon lime juice

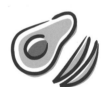

Blend the ingredients in a food processor or blender. This is a great dip for veggies, meat, or tofu bites, or a spread for sandwiches.

Sydney's green dip

- ½ cup plain yogurt
- ¼ cup frozen chopped spinach, thawed and drained

Blend. Some toddlers love this served alone! Swirl in extra yogurt for fun designs.

Speedy sesame sauce marinade

- 1 tablespoon grated fresh ginger
- 3 tablespoons tamari or soy sauce
- 1 teaspoon sesame oil
- 2 tablespoons honey

Remember, no honey for children less than one year old.

Whisk together ingredients and use the mixture to marinate chicken, fish, or tofu for one hour in the refrigerator, then grill or broil.

Creamy carrot spread

- 1 large carrot
- 4 ounces cream cheese
- 1 tablespoon orange juice
- ½ teaspoon cinnamon
- 1 teaspoon orange zest

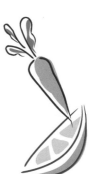

Thickly slice the carrot and boil or microwave in water until soft. Combine with the other ingredients using an electric blender or food processor.

Cheesy sauce

- 1 tablespoon butter
- 1 tablespoon all-purpose flour
- ¾ cup milk
- 1 cup grated Jack or cheddar cheese

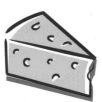

Melt the butter in a saucepan over gentle heat. Stir in the flour. Add milk. Cook and stir over medium heat until thickened. Add cheese and stir over low heat until melted. Great on pasta or veggies!

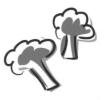

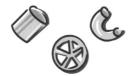

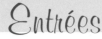
Honey-yogurt dip

- ½ cup plain yogurt
- 2 teaspoons apple cider vinegar
- 2 teaspoons honey

Remember, no honey for children less than one year old.

Mix and dip!

Grab & go's

If "mobile" describes your daily routine with your toddler, hopping between activities, child care, work, or play groups, you may choose to abandon all recipes and adopt this as your one and only snack list. Stock up on these foods for healthy, faster-than-fast-food munchies for toddlers on the move.

- Bite-sized dehydrated vegetable crisps
- Edamame (soybeans)
- Red bell pepper strips
- Frozen peas
- Fresh sliced or chopped fruit
- Raisin packs
- Dried fruit medleys
- Whole-grain fruit-sweetened cookies
- Rice cakes
- Goldfish crackers
- Dry low-sugar cereal
- Sliced nitrate-free turkey or soy "dogs"
- String cheese packets

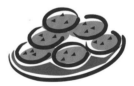

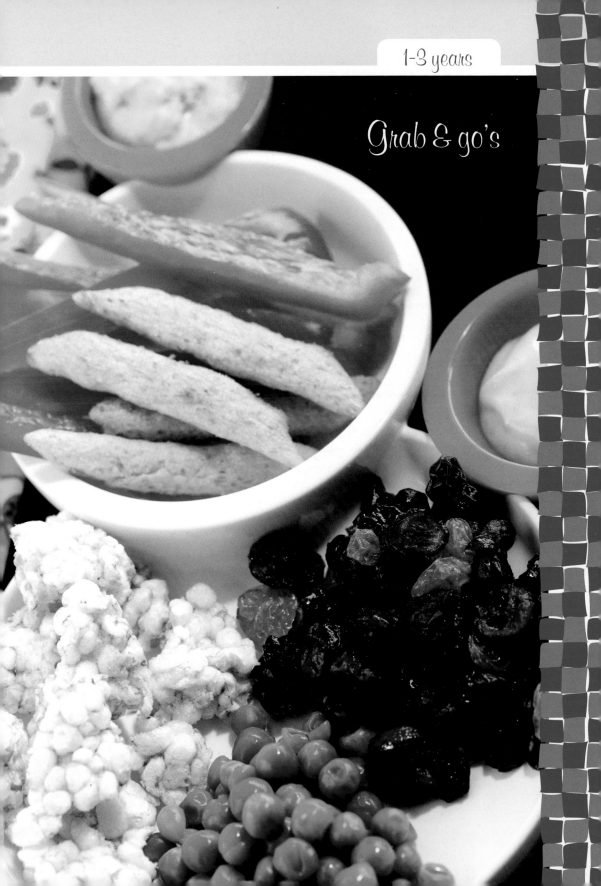

Grab & go's

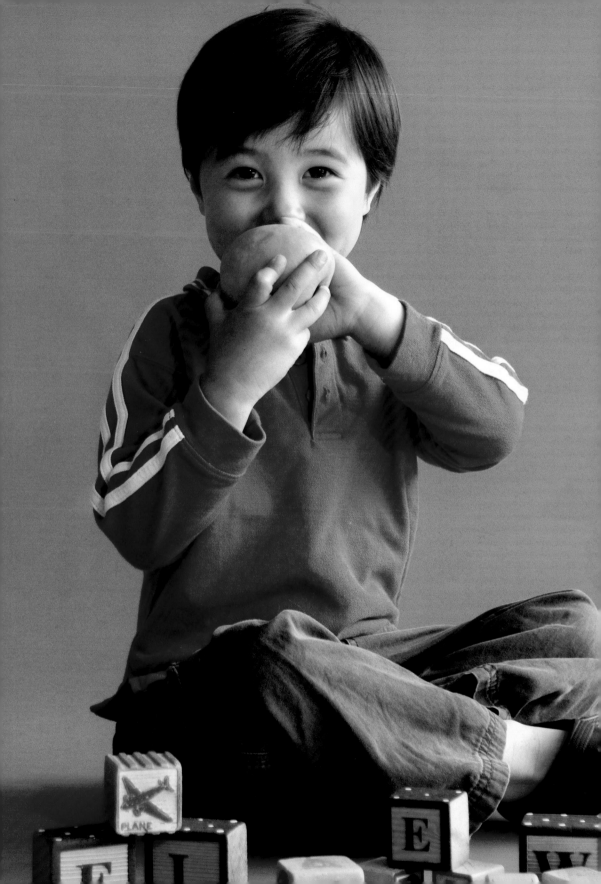

Á la Carte

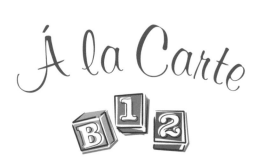

Stand out nutrients and supplement suggestions

he Toddler Bistro Á la Carte offers a carefully handpicked selection of valuable nutrients from carbohydrates to specific vitamins and minerals that are vital to your toddler's healthy development. I find that parents may have heard of a specific nutrient but are unsure of its function and why it is important. This chapter showcases some stand out toddler nutrients, lists recommended amounts, and offers a few supplement brand suggestions. My menu also offers a special side-order section for vegan families.

Á la Carte

As you stumble over questions about whether or not certain nutrients are important for your growing toddler, order up your answers from Á la Carte!

Notable nutrients

How do I know if my toddler is getting enough iron? Should I try to limit the amount of carbs he eats? My son won't drink milk, so what are some other good sources of calcium? Whether your nutrition knowledge brain fog is temporary or full time, these are common questions that I've addressed in this section, starting with big nutrient groups and then diving into the small ones.

Carbohydrates

Although carbohydrates are the diet buzzword of the twenty-first century, toddlers need them! Carbs are the brain's first choice for fuel. They get a bad rap because of "refining," how they are cooked, and overeating. More refined or processed foods generally contain fewer minerals, vitamins, and fiber, which leaves simple sugars, fat, and additives. Usually, the whiter the food, the more refined it is! Go for 100 percent whole grains in breads, rice, pasta, and cereals. Carbohydrates are also in beans, fruits, and vegetables, especially the starchy veggies like corn, potatoes, and peas.

Fiber

Fiber-rich foods even out blood sugar levels, feed our friendly intestinal bacteria, fight constipation (insoluble fiber) and diarrhea (soluble fiber), and contain many vitamins, minerals, and phytochemicals that help ward off chronic disease. Fiber is, however, filling and low in calories, and too much can prevent your toddler from getting enough energy. This may be more of a problem for vegan children (see Notable Nutrients for the Vegan Toddler, page 118).

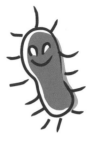

To calculate your child's daily fiber requirements, follow the suggestion of The American Academy of Pediatrics: Add 5 to your child's age. So for one-year-olds, fiber requirements equal 6 grams per day; for two-year-olds, figure on 7 grams per day, and so on.

Check this list for fabulous fiber-rich foods: **fruits, vegetables, beans, and grains**

- **Bran cereal:** ½ cup = 10.0 grams
- **Lentils:** ½ cup = 7.8 grams
- **Kidney beans:** ½ cup = 6.6 grams
- **Brown rice:** ½ cup = 5.3 grams
- **Acorn squash,** cooked: ½ cup = 5.3 grams
- **Apple:** 1 = 3.0 grams
- **Orange:** 1 = 2.9 grams
- **Broccoli,** cooked: ½ cup = 2.7 grams
- **Banana:** 1 = 2.5 grams
- **Oatmeal,** cooked: ½ cup = 2.2 grams
- **Carrot:** 1 = 2.1 grams

- **Oat bran**: 1 tablespoon = 2.0 grams
- **Wheat germ**: 1 tablespoon = 1.9 grams
- **Dried prunes**: 5 = 1.6 grams

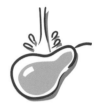

Make sure to wash and scrub all fruits and vegetables, especially the non-organic varieties.

Constipation concerns? If your toddler has the constipation blues, fiber may be both the cause and the cure. Fiber-rich foods that can be constipating are bananas, rice cereals, applesauce, carrots, and squash. Fiber-rich foods that help relieve constipation are pears, peaches, apricots, plums, beans, broccoli, whole grains, bran, and peas. Offering extra fluids may also help to ease constipation. Consult your health care provider if constipation is painful and prolonged.

Protein

Toddlers need protein for growth, tissue repair, muscles, hair, skin, hormones, healthy bones, and healthy immune systems. Protein also helps fight plaque buildup on teeth! Foods with a protein punch include meats, fish, and dairy products (find more sources in Notable Nutrients for the Vegan Toddler, page 118).

Check out this list for good sources of protein:

- 1 ounce roasted chicken breast = 9 grams
- 1 ounce beef (ground or steak) = 7 grams
- 1 ounce lean pork = 7 grams
- 1 ounce fish (halibut, salmon, flounder) = 6.5 grams
- 1 large egg = 6 grams

- 1 slice cheddar, American, or Swiss cheese = 7 grams
- 2 tablespoons Parmesan cheese = 12 grams
- ½ cup yogurt = 5 grams
- ½ cup milk = 4 grams

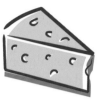

FYI: 2 cups of milk plus 1 ounce of meat are enough protein for a toddler's daily protein needs.

Fat

Fat stores energy, transports vitamins, and is very important for brain, central nervous system, and visual development. Our brains are 60 percent fat. In fact, during the first two years of life, the brain and central nervous system grow more than at any other time!

The skinny on fat is to make sure that saturated fats, found mostly in meat, whole-fat dairy, egg yolks, and palm and coconut oils, are only a very small portion of the diet. Favor unsaturated fats, especially the two "essential" fats, fats our bodies cannot make.

The two essential fats are:

1. **Linoleic (omega-6),** with a recommended daily intake of 7 grams. Sources are nuts, seeds, and vegetable and seed oils.

2. **Linolenic (omega-3),** with a recommended daily intake of 0.7 grams. Sources are flaxseeds, soybeans, walnuts, wheat germ, canola and flax oil, and fish, such as salmon, sardines, trout, catfish, and halibut (see First Course, Fishy Fish, page 29). The main omega-3 oil found in cold-water fish is DHA (see A Side of Supplements: DHA, page 127).

Most one- to two-year-olds do not get the necessary amounts of essential fats in their diet. Here's how to add healthy fats to your toddler's diet.

Add fabulous unsaturated foods such as avocados, walnuts, almonds, hazelnuts, flaxseeds, pumpkin seeds, sesame seeds, sunflower seeds, soybeans, and fish.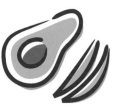

Use the following outstanding oils. For cooking, use canola, olive, soybean, or sesame oil. Add a tablespoon of oil to mashes, purées, and soups. You may add one or two tablespoons of flax, pumpkin, and walnut oil to foods after they are cooked or to cold foods and smoothies. Never use these oils for cooking: The heat destroys their wonderful benefits. The seeds and nuts that make these oils are fine to add to recipes.

Remember, avoid all products with trans fats, and wait on low-fat products until your toddler is two years old (see First Course, Foolish Fats, page 33).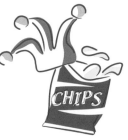

Calcium

Calcium is essential for strong bones and teeth! Only 50 percent of children ages one to five meet the recommended daily amount (RDA) for calcium, and it ranks as one of the most common nutrient deficiencies. Toddlers older than one year are at risk because their diet consists of more table food and less formula and breast milk. Healthy toddlers should be off formula at twelve months. Not to worry: One cup of milk plus one-half cup of yogurt will satisfy your toddler's daily calcium requirement.

Toddlers ages one to three years require 500 milligrams of calcium per day. Try these calcium-rich sources.

Toddler-sized foods that "got" calcium:

Chef's Tips

Always look for dairy products fortified with vitamin D. Among many other functions, we need this powerhouse vitamin to help maintain bone integrity!

- ½ cup plain yogurt = 225 milligrams
- 1 ounce cheddar cheese = 204 milligrams
- ½ cup milk = 150 milligrams
- 2 tablespoons dry nonfat milk = 104 milligrams
- ½ cup 2 percent cottage cheese = 76 milligrams
- 1 ounce canned salmon = 56 milligrams
- 1 ounce baked halibut = 17 milligrams

See Notable Nutrients for the Vegan Toddler, page 118, for nonanimal calcium sources.

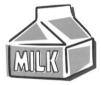

Iron

Red blood cells use iron to transport oxygen in our blood, which is vital to normal cognitive and physical development. Toddlers' brains grow rapidly during their first two years. They become more vulnerable to iron deficiency in their second year as their appetites fluctuate and they transition to cow's milk (which lacks iron, plus excessive amounts interfere with iron absorption). Iron-deficiency anemia is the most common nutritional problem for all children whether or not they eat meat. It has been associated with decreased learning, attention span, and motor and behavioral functioning.

These problems can be irreversible. Iron deficiency can also occur without anemia, and up to 30 percent of iron deficiency in toddlers may go undetected. To make a long story short, don't ignore the iron! Toddlers ages one to three years require 7 milligrams per day.

Serve these toddler-sized superb iron sources:

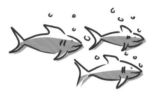

- 1 ounce pork = 1.1 milligrams
- 1 ounce beef = 1 milligram
- 1 large egg = 0.7 milligram
- 1 ounce poultry = 0.5 milligram
- 1 ounce lamb = 0.5 milligram
- 1 ounce fish = 0.3 milligram

See Notable Nutrients for the Vegan Toddler, below, for nonanimal iron sources.

Notable nutrients for the vegan toddler

Calcium and iron are very important for building healthy brains and bones for *all* toddlers, vegan or not! These minerals are easier to access from animal-based products, however, so check out the vegan food sources below to support your toddler's calcium and iron requirements.

Calcium

Calcium-fortified products are plentiful in today's market and are great options for vegan families. A variety of natural nonanimal sources of calcium are also available. If you make these foods a regular part of your toddler's menu, you should have no problem meeting the recommended 500 milligrams per day of calcium for your little plant-eater.

- ½ cup calcium-fortified soy milk = 150 milligrams
- 1 tablespoon blackstrap molasses = 137 milligrams
- ½ cup calcium-fortified regular tofu = 130 milligrams
- ½ cup cooked soybeans = 90 milligrams
- ½ cup boiled bok choy = 80 milligrams
- 2 tablespoons almonds = 80 milligrams
- 1 corn tortilla = 50 milligrams
- ½ cup cooked kale = 47 milligrams
- ½ cup cooked or fresh broccoli = 45 milligrams
- ½ medium orange = 26 milligrams
- ½ slice whole wheat bread = 16 milligrams

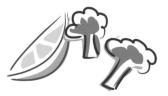

Chef's Tips

Look for milk substitutes that offer 30 percent of the daily value (DV) for calcium and that are fortified with vitamin D.

Oxalic acid binds up the calcium in spinach, chard, beet greens, and rhubarb, preventing absorption. Other dark green leafies (broccoli, kale, collards) are good calcium sources.

Iron

Iron is quite prominent in the plant kingdom, although it comes in a form that is harder for us to absorb than iron from meats. Some experts suggest that vegans should aim for a higher amount of daily iron than the recommended 7 milligrams per day for omnivores.

Foods common to the vegan diet, however, are solid sources of iron, as you see from the list of iron-power edibles below.

- ½ cup 100 percent fortified, ready-to-eat cereal = 9 grams
- 1 tablespoon blackstrap molasses = 5 milligrams
- ½ cup cooked soybeans = 4 grams
- ½ cup fortified oatmeal = 4 grams
- ½ cup cooked lentils = 3 grams
- ½ cup cooked fresh spinach = 3 grams
- ½ cup refried beans = 2.5 milligrams
- ½ cup tofu = 1.8 grams
- 2 tablespoons peanut butter = 1.1 milligrams
- 2 tablespoons cashews = 1 milligram
- 1 slice bread or ½ bagel = 1 milligram
- ½ cup soymilk = 0.9 milligram
- 2 tablespoons dried apricots = 0.8 milligram
- 2 tablespoons raisins = 0.5 milligram
- ½ cup mashed potatoes = 0.3 milligram
- 1 kiwi = 0.3 milligram

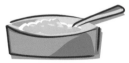

Chef's Tips

Iron from meats, poultry, and fish is more easily absorbed by humans than iron from plant sources. Vitamin C foods and foods high in protein increase iron absorption. If you have a famous spaghetti sauce recipe, try cooking it in a cast-iron pot. This is another way to add iron to your veggie-based foods.

Multivitamins/minerals with iron are also helpful (see A Side of Supplements, page 123).

Vitamin B12

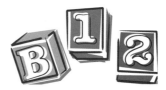

Vitamin B12 is important for growth and nerve development. Because B12 is found mainly in animal products, milk, and dairy, it is virtually absent in the vegan diet. Additionally, vegan diets are high in folate, which can mask a B12 deficiency. Vitamin B12 deficiencies manifest as megaloblastic anemia, and some progress to irreversible nerve damage. Vegan B12 food sources are fortified foods, Red Star nutritional yeast, meat substitutes, and some cooked sea vegetables such as hijiki and wakame. A daily multivitamin/mineral containing B12 is a good idea to help boost your toddler's intake.

Toddlers from one to three years of age require 0.9 micrograms per day.

Zinc

Zinc aids in normal growth and development and boosts the immune system. Zinc is routinely administered to third-world infants and children to help improve growth and to combat diarrhea and lower-respiratory infections. Zinc is best absorbed from meats, fish, dairy, and eggs. Although zinc is also in whole grains and beans, these foods contain "phytates," which can bind it and block absorption. Vegan foods that help zinc absorption are yeast-leavened breads and fermented soy products such as miso, tamari, or tempeh.

Toddlers from one to three years of age require 3 milligrams of zinc per day.

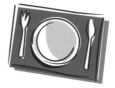

Serve these toddler-sized zinc sources:

- 2 tablespoons Red Star nutritional yeast = 3.2 grams
- ½ cup bran flakes = 2.5 milligrams
- 2 tablespoons wheat germ = 2.3 milligrams
- 1 tablespoon tahini = 1.6 milligrams
- ½ cup chickpeas (garbanzo beans) = 1.3 milligrams
- ½ cup tofu = 1 milligram

Protein

Providing protein-rich foods for vegan toddlers requires extra attention, because most plant foods do not contain all nine of the essential amino acids found in meats, fish, or dairy protein. "Essential" means that we can't make them, and we need amino acids to make proteins! The trick is to serve grains and beans (they do not have to be served at the same meal) during the day to equal a full protein. The plant family does have a few exceptions that offer all of the essential amino acids: soy foods, quinoa (actually a seed), amaranth, and buckwheat.

Choose from these protein-power vegan foods:

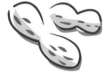

- 2 tablespoons peanut butter = 10 grams
- ½ cup cooked soybeans = 10 grams
- ½ cup refried beans = 9 grams
- 2 tablespoons Red Star nutritional yeast = 8.3 grams
- ½ cup cooked split peas = 8 grams
- ½ cup cooked beans (lentils, black, kidney, pinto, garbanzo) = 7 grams
- 2 tablespoons chopped walnuts = 7 grams
- ½ cup tofu = 6.5 grams
- 2 tablespoons slivered almonds = 5 grams
- ½ cup soy milk = 3.3 grams
- ½ cup cooked spinach = 3 grams
- 1 slice whole wheat bread = 2.7 grams
- ½ cup cooked rice = 2.5 grams
- ½ cup mashed potatoes = 2 grams
- ½ cup broccoli = 2 grams

A side of supplements

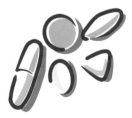

It is easy to go overboard when considering the wide array of supplements available in today's market. I have seen some people's cabinets that harbor a figurative tackle box full of various powders and capsules that look like they are ingredients for a cauldron of brew rather than simply a boost for a normal, healthy diet. As a nutritionist, I always preach getting the bulk of nutrients from the actual food rather than using nutritional supplements as an excuse to eat candy and French fries. So, what about for your toddler? Is a multivitamin necessary?

The multivitamins/minerals montage

Multivitamins/minerals can help to fill in those nutritional gaps caused by toddlers' erratic appetites and crazy food preferences. Liquids are available for teeth-challenged toddlers and chewables for toddlers with molars. Nature is still the best package for the vitamins and minerals we know about—and those we don't—so supplements are no substitute for a healthy, balanced diet. They are simply a good insurance policy. Chewables taste good, so store them out of reach and eyesight of your tempted toddler!

The Toddler Bistro's favorite multivitamin recipe

If you want to hunt down a toddler multivitamin/mineral, photocopy these tables to take with you to the store. The first section lists the recommended dietary amounts of vitamins for toddlers one to three years old, and the second section lists recommended amounts of minerals. Remember, this is an ideal list, and most brands will not have an exact match. If you find most of these on the label, you are in good shape. Make sure that the serving size isn't eight tablets a day! For a shortcut to some brand suggestions, flip to Toddler Bistro Bests, page 127.

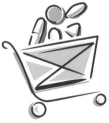

VITAMIN	FORM	RDA
A	beta-carotene	3,000 IUs
	retinyl palmitate	990 IUs
C	ascorbic acid, ester-C	15 mg
D	D3, cholecalciferol, ergocalciferol	400 IUs*
E	d-alpha-tocopherol or mixed tocopherols	9 IUs
K	phylloquinone	30 µg
B1	thiamin	0.5 mg
B2	riboflavin	0.5 mg
B3	niacin	6 mg
B5	pantothenic acid	2 mg
B6	pyridoxine, pyridoxal-5-phosphate	0.5 mg
Folic Acid	folic acid, folate	150 µg
B12	methylcobalamin	0.9 µg
Biotin	biotin, biocytin	8 µg

Caution! *If your vitamin A is listed as retinol or retinyl palmitate, this is the fat-soluble form that can accumulate in the body. Toxicity has only been observed at extremely high doses—at least ten times the RDA. Avoid cod liver oil, which naturally contains high levels of retinol.*

*Recommended by the American Academy of Pediatrics

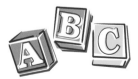

125

MINERAL	FORM	RDA/AI
Calcium	calcium citrate, malate, carbonate	500 mg
Magnesium	magnesium citrate	80 mg
Potassium	potassium citrate, aspartate	3000 mg
Iron	ferrous succinate, sulfate	7 mg
Zinc	zinc aspartate, citrate	3 mg
Copper	copper sulfate, picolinate	340 µg
Chromium	chromium glycinate, picolinate	11 µg
Selenium	selenomethionine	20 ug
Manganese	manganese, amino acid chelate	1.2 mg
Fluoride		0.7 mg
Molybdenum	molybdenum, amino acid chelate	17 µg
Phosphorus		460 mg
Iodine	potassium iodide	90 µg
OTHER		
Choline	choline bitartrate	200 mg

FYI: *Iron fights zinc and calcium absorption, so make sure that you are serving calcium-rich foods. Vitamin C foods help in iron absorption, while fibrous foods can interfere. Zinc's availability also decreases with fiber, as well as with iron and calcium. Protein and milk help zinc absorption. All of this means that there is no substitute for a healthy diet!*

The Toddler Bistro's multivitamin/mineral Bistro Bests:

- **Rainbow Light Kids' One** (Santa Cruz, California)
  These are easy one-a-day chewables. This brand does leave out choline, and is a little low on zinc, iron, magnesium, and calcium, but it is still one of the best available.

- **Centrum Kids Complete Chewable Multivitamin** (Madison, New Jersey)
  Serve one-half tablet a day. The only nutrients this chewable is missing are selenium and choline! This brand does contain aspartame, in case your toddler needs to avoid this sweetener.

- **Natural Factors Big Friends Chewables** (Canada)
  Another great one-a-day chewable. Big Friends has all the necessary nutrients, although it is under the RDA for magnesium, iron, zinc, and choline.

DHA

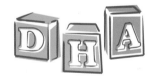

DHA (docosahexanoic acid) is an omega-3 fatty acid that is vital to brain, eye, and central nervous system development from prebirth through the first two years of life. In fact, it is the most abundant fatty acid in the brain! DHA is included in several formulas and is naturally contained in breast milk. Food sources are primarily cold-water fish, such as salmon, trout, or sardines, and fortified eggs. As you wean your toddlers from formula or breast milk, it is likely that their DHA intake will diminish, especially if you are raising them as vegans or do not serve fish regularly (two to three times per week).

DHA supplements come in capsule or liquid form, either fish oil–based or algae-grown. You can mix the oil into a smoothie or yogurt. More tasty, fruit-flavored varieties are also available. Your toddler may decide that algae-grown is more palate-pleasing than the fish oil brands.

Aim for 100 milligrams per day for children from birth to two years of age.

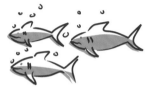

The Toddler Bistro's Bests:

- **Carlson for Kids Chewable DHA** (Arlington Heights, Illinois)
  Orange-flavored fish oil, 100-milligram capsules

- **Source Naturals DHA** (Scotts Valley, California)
  Algae-grown, 100-milligram capsules

- **Nature's Way Neuromins** (Springville, Utah)
  Plant-sourced DHA, 100-milligram capsules

Probiotics and prebiotics

Probiotics, meaning "pro-life," (*bifidobacteria*, L. *acidophilus*, L. *bulgaricus*, L. *rhamnosus*, L. *thermophilus*) are the friendly bacteria living in our intestines. Prebiotics, such as fructooligosaccharides (FOS) and inulin, are derived from nondigestible fiber and function to enhance the growth of these healthy bacteria.

Studies link probiotics with many benefits, such as improving intestinal tract health, limiting lactose intolerance and food allergy reactions, making nutrients, increasing nutrient absorption, and strengthening the immune system by fighting off disease-causing bacteria. Food sources are milk, yogurt, and kefir (fermented milk).

If your toddler is prone to infections, allergic dermatitis, or diarrhea, you may want to consider a probiotics supplement (see Toddler Bistro Bests, below).

The shelf life of refrigerated products is about three to six weeks; for dried supplements, it's approximately twelve months.

Probiotics are not yet FDA approved. Consult your health care provider.

Be a "CLR" (compulsive label reader) for the Live & Active Cultures seal on dairy products.

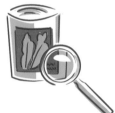

Toddler Bistro Bests:

- **Baby's Jarro-Dophilus, Jarrow Formulas** (Canada)
  This is a powder containing bifidobacteria and lactobacilli with fructooligosaccharides (FOS), 3 billion cultures per gram (¼ teaspoon). Look for this in the refrigerated section of health food stores. It should be given with food either by putting ¼ teaspoon on your toddler's tongue with a meal or snack, or mixed into food or a beverage.

- **Nature's Way Primadophilus for Children or Kids** (Springville, Utah)
  This product is offered in powder or chewable tablets and should be given with food. One serving contains bifidobacteria and lactobacilli, 1 billion microorganisms per tablet.

- **Nutrition Now Rhino FOS and Acidophilus**
  (Vancouver, Washington)
  This product is offered in powder or chewable tablets. One serving contains 1 billion bifidobacteria and lactobacilli and should be given with food.

Protein powders

Protein powders make toddlers' digestive systems do a lot of work, may impair absorption of other amino acids, and provide only small amounts of protein in comparison to foods. In other words, they should be avoided! If you think your toddler needs to gain weight, add extra calories and consult your health care provider (see Extras, Weight Worries, page 138).

Herbs

If you want to give your toddler herbal supplements, please realize that they are formulated in doses intended for druglike effects. Toddlers' livers are not fully developed and may not be able to filter herbs at an adult pace. Herbs may also cause allergies and interact with other medications, so consult your health care provider before you use them!

Teaching toddlers about nutrients

It's fun to teach toddlers about the nutrients in foods and how they keep us healthy. Most of us know that milk builds solid bones, but there is more! Use this table as a learning tool to talk to your toddler about how foods help our bodies function at their best.

VITAMIN	HEALTH BENEFIT	FOOD SOURCE
A	eyes, skin, immune system	meat, egg yolk, dairy, yellow and orange carotenoids, dark green, leafy veggies, cantaloupe, peaches, apricots
D	bones, teeth, calcium absorption	D-fortified milk, fish, egg yolk, liver, sunlight (10 to 15 minutes, two to three times per week)
E	fights cell damage, immune system	vegetable oils, wheat germ, nuts, egg yolk, dark green leafies, milk fat
K	blood clotting, bones	vegetable oils, dark green leafies, wheat bran, "friendly" intestinal bacteria make it
Thiamin	growth, energy usage	beans, liver, enriched grains
Riboflavin	growth	milk, dairy, eggs, liver, dark green leafies, enriched grains
Niacin	energy usage	fish, meat, poultry, liver, grains, beans, eggs, peanuts
B6	growth	pork, liver, bran, milk, egg yolk, beans, oatmeal
Folate	nervous system, red blood cells, DNA	dark green leafies, meat, liver, fish, wheat, eggs, beans, yeast

B12	nervous system, growth, red blood cells	milk, dairy, meat, liver, eggs, poultry
Pantothenic acid	energy usage	eggs, liver, salmon, yeast, all plant and animal foods
Biotin	maintains proteins and fats	liver, fruits, veggies, peanuts, yeast, meat, milk, egg yolk, "friendly" intestinal bacteria make it
C	immune system, wound healing, iron absorption	citrus, kiwis, strawberries, tomatoes, greens, peppers

MINERAL	HEALTH BENEFIT	FOOD SOURCE
Calcium	bones, teeth, muscles, nerves	milk, dairy, sardines, dark leafies, tofu
Phosphorus	bones, teeth, energy	milk, meat, poultry, fish, grains, beans, nuts
Sodium	stable cells, fluid balance	everything!
Chloride magnesium	bones, muscles, energy, stable cells, stomach acid	grains, tofu, nuts, green veggies, beans, table salt, fish, milk, meat, eggs
Potassium	stable cells, energy use	fruits, veggies, cereals, milk, meat, beans

Iron	red blood cells, oxygen transport	meat, egg yolk, beans, dark green veggies, shellfish, dark molasses
Zinc	growth, immune system, healing	shellfish, milk, liver, beans, wheat bran
Copper	energy, immune system, tissues	shellfish, liver, grains, beans, poultry, nuts, cherries
Chromium	blood sugar balance	grains, meats, yeast, clams
Selenium	immune system, fat usage	grains, onions, milk, meats, veggies
Manganese	tissue, energy usage	blueberries, grains, beet greens, nuts, beans
Fluoride	bones, teeth	drinking water, rice, soybeans, greens, onions
Molybdenum	protein reactions	beans, grains, dark leafies, liver
Iodine	thyroid, cell energy	iodized table salt, seafood, water, veggies
OTHER		
Choline	nervous system, brain development	eggs, milk, liver, soybeans, beef, peanuts, kale, cabbage

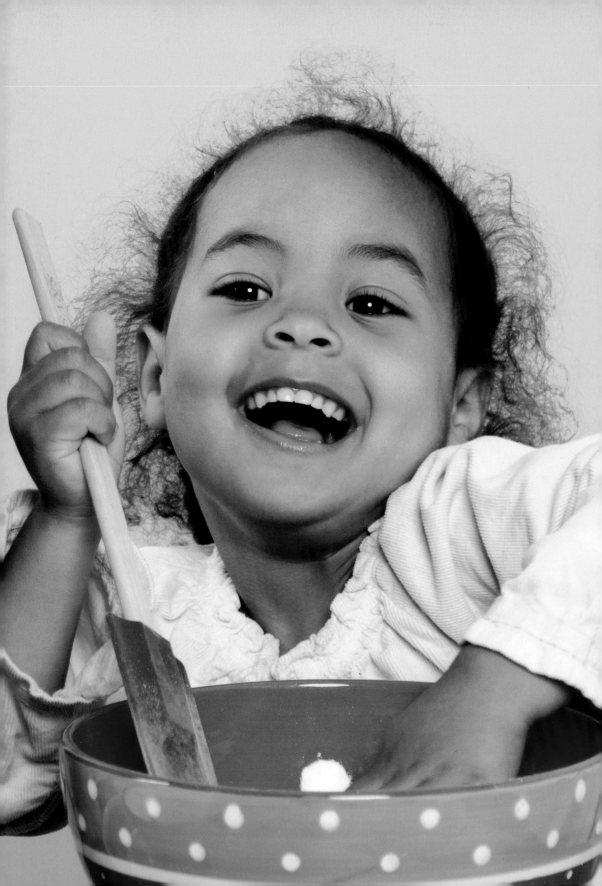

Extras

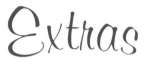

Taming today's trends

The Toddler Bistro Extras is a panache of pointers for parents on how to tackle some common nutrition-related topics with today's toddlers. Life moves quickly, and it is easy to slip into unhealthy habits as a convenience or simply as an oversight. Most times, though, these habits are harder to undo the longer we let them last. Whether you have concerns about your child's weight or whether his or her television viewing is careening out of control, pay a little attention now, and build a healthier future for your toddler and family.

Digesting the facts on fast food

Okay . . . let's face it—most of us succumb to fast food at some point. It tastes good, it's easy, and it comes with toys—what a combination! But, guess what? French fries *are not* a healthy vegetable choice! Research has revealed that the number-one veggie for one- to two-year-olds is fries, and that more than half of two- to three-year-olds don't get enough daily fruits and veggies.

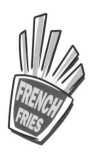

It's no surprise that toddlers who eat fast food regularly have higher intakes of fat, salt, cholesterol, and calories and lower intakes of vitamins, minerals, and fiber. Fast food serving sizes are four to six times the sizes they were in 1955! The average chocolate chip cookie has grown in size by 700 percent. Size aside, common methods of cooking popular dishes in fast food restaurants and by snack food manufacturers are not so great either. Research has found that frying, grilling, or baking starchy foods (fries, potato chips, cookies) forms a chemical called acrylamide, a "probable" human carcinogen according to the World Health Organization. This is one more reason to skip those greasy French fries and potato chips in the family meals!

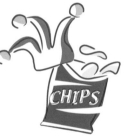

Follow these Bistro Basics to control fast food in your toddler's diet:

- Don't make fast food a habit. Fast food is acceptable on occasion, but only in moderation.
- When you do go, avoid the battered, creamy, buttery, fried, cheesy, saucy, salty, and giant-sized selections.

- Choose grilled, skinless, steamed, broiled, roasted, baked, thin crusts, lots of vegetables, and low-sodium sauces. Soy, teriyaki, barbecue sauce, and gravy are high in sodium.
- Remember, toddler-sized servings! (See Starters: Four-star Fundamentals, page 12.)
- If the toy in the meal is the big attraction for your toddler, try adding a toy or stickers to your own healthy creation in a fun container or brightly colored bag and call it a "Merry Meal."

Television time

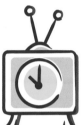

The American Academy of Pediatrics recommends *no TV* for toddlers younger than two years of age. Toddlers older than two may watch one to two hours per day. Some research shows that even two hours of TV a day increase the risk for obesity among two- to five-year-olds. Restricting TV may be difficult, but remember that you are building your toddler's imagination, creativity, and self-sufficiency skills. They can live without satellite or cable!

For toddlers two years old and older

In the majority of families, some toddler TV time is inevitable, and yes, I know, it can be a welcome break for tired moms. Try some TV monitoring techniques. Show select screenings to your toddlers. Allow them to choose from educational TV programming and age-appropriate videos or DVDs.

Aim for commercial-free TV. Young children watch commercials with the same attention level as they watch their TV shows, and they don't discern between the two. Research indicates that it takes two- to six-year-olds only a couple of times of watching a ten- to thirty-second commercial to influence their food product preferences. Since most food commercials during children's programming advertise fatty, sugary, and salty foods, you are in danger of having a little junk food junkie on your hands if you do not cut out commercials.

Be the TV master. Decide when and how much TV, and turn it on and off for the chosen show.

Let TV time follow active play. Try a toddler activity video or fitness video game, too! Toddlers love programs where they participate by dancing or moving along with fun characters or animals and music.

Make meals TV-free! Children in families who watch TV with two meals a day eat more fast food, pizza, salty snacks, and soda and fewer fruits and veggies. Without TV, diet and mealtime behavior improve.

Weight worries

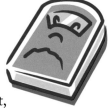

Overweight and obese children are a growing international concern. Almost 14 percent of two- to five-year-olds in the United States are overweight, and one in three is at risk for becoming overweight. In addition, these children are more likely to develop chronic diseases, such as diabetes, some cancers, osteoarthritis, and high blood pressure, as well as be overweight as adults.

Learn about the dangers of obesity. Consult with your health care professional to help you determine your toddler's body mass index (BMI), or calculate it online, using the online BMI calculator (http://pediatrics.about.com/cs/usefultools/l/bl_bmi_calc.htm). A BMI at or higher than 95 percent is considered overweight. BMI is calculated from height and weight and is not a measure of body fat. For example, a BMI indicating that a child is overweight may not be an accurate measure for a large-boned, muscular child with normal body fat.

The National Institutes of Health (NIH) defines overweight as body weight that is more than 20 percent of the recommended weight. Toddlers who may be more at risk are those with one or both parents who are obese, were low birth weight infants, are inactive, watch a lot of TV (see Television Time, page 137), and eat mostly fatty and fast foods (see Digesting the Facts on Fast Food, page 136).

Studies show that moms often misinterpret their toddlers' hunger cues, and some cultures believe that chubby children are healthier. On the contrary, overweight toddlers are in greater danger of developing chronic diseases. They also battle peer ridicule and poor self-esteem.

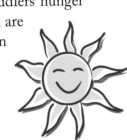

Follow these tips to chase away the chubbies:

- No diets! Concentrate on healthy foods and weight maintenance, and let your toddler's growth catch up to his or her weight.
- Reinforce healthy eating with praise and role modeling.
- Avoid frequent fast food trips and high calorie drinks. Juice, soda, and too much milk (more than 24 ounces per day) can add a significant amount of calories to your child's daily energy intake.

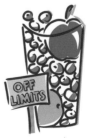

- Don't supersize servings (see Starters, Four-star Fundamentals, page 12).
- Trade in TV time for physical activity. Each hour of TV viewing boosts the chances of becoming obese.
- Family-based behavioral changes make healthy habits last longer.
- Food is fuel, not a tool in the chest of bribes, rewards, punishments, and threats. Rather than having to clean their plate or be on good behavior for a candy bar, toddlers need to learn to listen to their bodies' signals for hunger and fullness. Using food to mold behavior robs your toddler of this essential ability.
- Babysitters and day care facilities should have activities and healthy snacks planned.

Menu checks

Here are some menu tricks to trim the fat and calories without introducing a weight-loss diet. The goal is to stop weight gain, not to force weight loss. Weight loss may be unhealthy for developing children.

- Dairy (for toddlers older than two years): Serve skim or 1 percent milk, nonfat yogurt, nonfat sour cream, and nonfat evaporated skim milk instead of cream. Serve cheeses like Parmesan, mozzarella, and Swiss, which are lower in fat and calories. Talk to your health care provider about serving low-fat dairy if your toddler is under two years of age.
- Substitute canola oil, olive oil, salsa, spices, vinegar- or citrus-based dressings, cooking sprays, and chicken or vegetable broths for butter, shortening, and margarine.

- Spread sandwiches with tomato sauce or paste, mustard, ketchup, or veggie purées.
- Use egg whites instead of the whole egg (2 egg whites = 1 whole egg in recipes).
- Bake, broil, grill, or poach meats and fish instead of frying them.
- Trim fat, remove skin, and drain fat from meat sautés.
- Choose lean meats, poultry, fish, and beans.
- Stay clear of sugary foods and drinks. (see First Course, Summing Up Salt, Sugar, and Spice, page 35.)

Underweight? Consult your health care provider if you think your toddler is underweight. Reasons for low body weight are lack of appetite alone, or poor appetite caused by illness, constipation, diarrhea, stress, or inadequate nutrient absorption.

Use this Menu Checklist to bulk up your toddler:

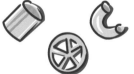

- Add extra calories to your toddler's daily diet. Offer whole-fat dairy products and include healthy, nutrient-dense foods, such as nut butters, starchy veggies, pasta, breads, yogurts, cheeses, dried fruits, and cereals.
- Fat intake should be 30 percent of daily calories (see Notable Nutrients, Fat, page 115).
- Establish regular mealtimes, and make sure to include snacks. Your goal should be three meals a day with two to three snacks.
- Serve your toddler's favorites!
- Fill in nutrient gaps with a daily multivitamin/mineral (see Á la Carte, A Side of Supplements, page 123).

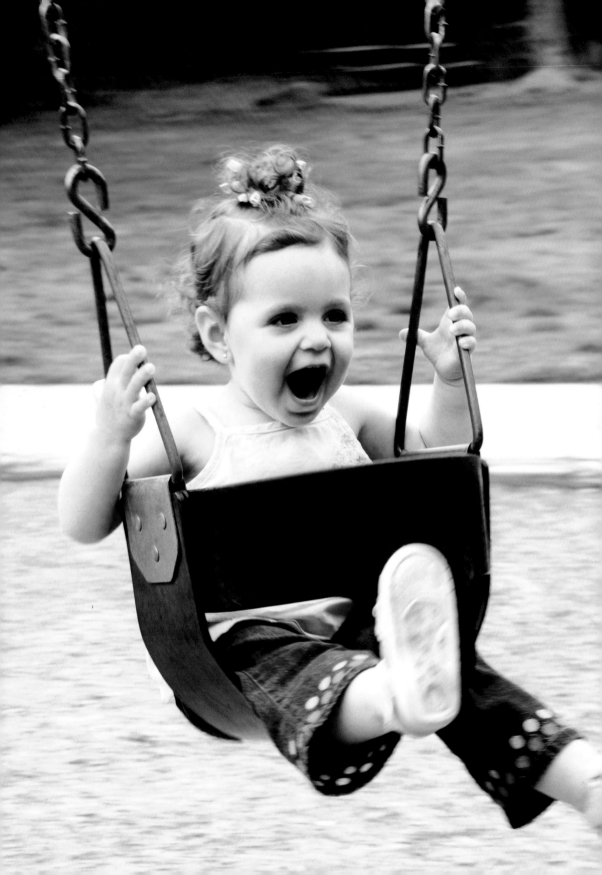

Desserts

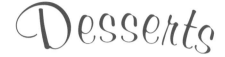

Healthy habits for life

Serving nutritious foods is just a skip down the path to establishing the foundation for a healthy lifestyle for your toddler. What is the recipe for a healthy child? Alas, the dessert ingredients below are not for the best brownie in the world, but they will help raise a blue-ribbon healthy toddler.

The Toddler Bistro

Fitness special features

Oh where, oh where did physical activity go? That time is getting devoured by the computer, television, and video game monsters. A sedentary lifestyle is a major factor, along with fast food and super serving sizes, in the current obesity crisis. Digital games that do not involve physical activity and computers for toddlers may be educational and are fine in moderation but should be balanced with outdoor and indoor active play.

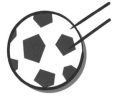

The National Association of Sports and Physical Education (NASPE) recommends that toddlers have at least thirty minutes a day of structured physical activity and sixty minutes a day of unstructured free play. It may tire you out, but outside of sleeping, toddlers should be active most of the day and should not be idle for more than an hour at a time. Research shows that prolonged inactivity can lead to obesity and delay development of movement skills. So, keep intermissions brief! For more information, visit www.aahperd.org.

Day care programs and babysitters need to have activities planned other than watching videos! Ask your day care coordinators about how they structure their program. Talk with your babysitter about safe outdoor or indoor active play. My favorites were walks with "I Spy" and rainy day "Follow the Leader" games.

The next Olympic gold may or may not be in your toddler's future, but here are some basic rewards that he or she will gain from regular exercise:

- Establishes a healthy habit.
- Builds toddlers' motor skills, coordination, and concentration.

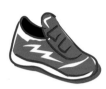

- Increases toddlers' self-confidence and the sense of control of their bodies.
- Lessens the chances of becoming overweight.
- Provides family bonding time.

Family sweets

Fostering your toddler's interest in nutritious foods stems from everyday experiences at home with family and caretakers. "Family sweets" are tried-and-true generational secrets to enjoying time with your children and simultaneously sparking their awareness of healthy food choices.

Create an ongoing story with your toddler and add to it at bedtime, during quiet time, or on car rides. Use new words like "leaping" lettuce or "slippery" squash.

Bath time can be fun and inspire learning. Trace shapes of what you are serving or served for dinner on your toddler's back, and have him or her guess what it is. Your child may be more excited to eat that food!

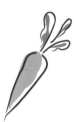

Flip pages in a magazine with your toddler, looking for foods from a food group like fruits or grains, and create a cuisine collage!

Create a recipe together. Set up a step stool at the counter and have your toddlers help you stir, wash fruits and veggies, or pour in measured amounts. Make faces on mini-pizzas or cookies with veggies or raisins. Even if they don't eat it, at least you inspired some creativity and helped them build kitchen confidence!

Desserts

Make your kitchen the gathering place for family fun. Many recipes are handed down over generations and are like diaries for families. Learning the basics of good health and nutrition is that secret extra ingredient.

Develop family traditions for holidays or special occasions. My job was always to stir the Thanksgiving gravy as a child, and it remains my specialty to this day. Holidays are wonderful opportunities to help your children become comfortable in the kitchen, cooking recipes.

Make simple picnics and have your toddler help find just the right spot to enjoy your outdoor dining! Older toddlers can help choose and prepare healthy selections for the picnic. Pack it up in a fun, colorful container. Your children may surprise you and try that piece of broccoli that they typically reject. Everything tastes better outside!

Draw pictures together of a fruit or vegetable and make up a story like "The Adventures of the Monkey and the Banana" or "The Spaghetti and the Giant Tomato." Talk about how the foods are healthy while you draw and then frame your little Picasso's artwork for room decoration. Make your story ongoing to continue during quiet times, car rides, or bedtime.

Celebrate your toddler time. You will never get it back.

---

*Three years old,
a joy to behold.
My love for you,
forever unfolds.*

Appendix 1

A spoonful of sources

I thought I would spare you from the piles of clinical research studies and twenty-pound textbooks in my office. However, you may enjoy perusing a sampling of other books and online resources from my home library. Throughout the book I refer to many Web sites, so I have listed them again here for easier access. Let the learning begin!

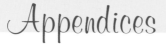
Books

Dowshen, Steven A., M.D. *Fit Kids*. New York: DK Publishing Inc., 2004.

Joneja, Janice Vickerstaff, PhD, R.D. *Dealing with Food Allergies in Babies and Children*. Boulder, Colo.: Bull Publishing Company, 2007.

Kleinman, Ronald E., M.D. *Pediatric Nutrition Handbook*, 5th ed. Elk Grove Village, Ill.: American Academy of Pediatrics, 2004.

Tamborlane, William V., M.D. *The Yale Guide to Children's Nutrition*. New Haven, Conn.: Yale University Press, 1994.

Ward, Elizabeth M., M.S., R.D. *Healthy Foods, Healthy Kids*. Avon, Mass.: Adams Media Corporation, 2002.

Web sites

Children's health and nutrition
www.aap.org
www.babycenter.com
www.mypyramid.gov
www.nih.gov
www.parenting.ivillage.com
To determine Body Mass Index:
    http://pediatrics.about.com/cs/
    usefultools/l/bl_bmi_calc.htm

Drinking water safety
www.epa.gov/safewater
www.leadtesting.org/orderonline.htm
My Water's Fluoride: http://apps.
    nccd.cdc.gov/MWF/Index.asp
www.nsf.org

Environmental safety
www.cdc.gov
www.consumersunion.org
www.cspinet.org/nah/bpa.html
www.epa.gov/lead
www.fsis.usda.gov/factsheets/
    cooking_safely_in_the_
    microwave/index.asp
www.epa.gov/smokefree/
www.iatp.org
www.ewg.org

Food additives
www.cspinet.org/reports/
    chemcuisine.htm

Food allergies
www.celiac.org
www.foodallergy.org
www.kidswithfoodallergies.org

Seafood safety
www.fda.gov/Food/FoodSafety/
    Product-SpecificInformation/
    Seafood/FoodbornePathogens
    Contaminants/Methylmercury/
    ucm115644.htm
www.eatwellguide.org/search.cfm
www.edf.org
www.epa.gov/waterscience/fish

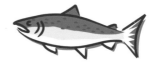

Appendix 2
Shopping simplicity

ere is my "if I were you at the market" section. Not all of these brands will be available in your area. Flip to First Course, Shopping Smarts, page 37, for general shopping guidelines to help you select healthy food brands.

Appendices

Bread section

Tortillas and pita

Buenatural organic whole wheat tortillas

Garden of Eatin' organic pita breads, whole wheat tortillas, organic chapati

La Tortilla Factory organic whole wheat tortillas

Trader Joe's organic whole wheat and corn flour tortillas, handmade corn tortillas, whole wheat pita

Tumaro's Gourmet Tortillas (garden spinach and vegetables, honey wheat)

Whole Foods 365 Organic Tortillas (whole wheat, traditional)

Breads

Arnold Natural 100 percent whole wheat oat, 100 percent whole wheat

EarthGrains honey whole grains

Healthy Choice honey wheat, soy and flaxseed, hearty 100 percent whole grain

Millbrook 100 percent whole wheat

Milton's healthy whole grain, gourmet white, potato

Nature's Own 100 percent whole wheat

Oroweat health nut original

Pepperidge Farm natural whole grain, Farmhouse 100 percent whole wheat

Sara Lee cinnamon raisin swirl mini-bagels, heart-healthy whole wheat bagels, 100 percent whole wheat, sliced

Trader Joe's almost whole wheat pizza dough, refrigerated, whole-grain English muffins, fat-free English muffins, wheat mini-bagels, sprouted wheat cinnamon raisin bagels mini-bran muffins with raisins, sprouted barley, Pilgrim's Harvest molasses multigrain

Vogel mixed whole grain

Cereal section

Arrowhead Mills flakes, instant oatmeal (original plain or seven-grain), Health Valley organic oat bran O's, organic raisin bran flakes

Back to Nature Hi-Protein Crunch cereal

Barbara's Bakery Puffins (original, honey rice, cinnamon), Organic Wild Puffs

Cascadian Farms Organic Purley O's, Honey Nut O's, raisin bran, multi-grain squares

Country Choice organic oven-toasted oats

EnviroKidz Organic Gorilla Munch cereal

General Mills Cheerios

Kashi Heart to Heart honey toasted oat cereal, Go Lean Crunch, Puffed Kashi

Malt-O-Meal

Mother's 100 percent natural rolled oats, hot rolled whole wheat cereal

Naturally Preferred Organic raisin bran

Nature's Path organic multigrain oat bran and raisins, Organic Flax Plus raisin bran, Organic Heritage O's multigrain, instant hot oatmeal—original Old Wessex Ltd. 100 percent instant hot cereals

Quaker Oats

Trader Joe's oat bran flakes with raisins, Oatmeal Complete

Whole Foods 365 raisin bran, whole oat O's

Whole Kids organic cereal Morning-O's, Honey Nut Morning-O's, Rainbow Rings

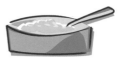

Pasta section

Dried pastas

Annie's Homegrown organic microwavable macaroni and cheese, shells and white cheddar, whole wheat shells and cheddar
Davinci shells, wagon wheels, bowties
De Boles organic pastas
DeCecco pasta tricolor bows
Delverde organic pastas
Eddie's organic soy penne, vegetable bowties
Eden's organic pastas
Hodgson Mill organic pastas
Mrs. Leepers organic pastas
Trader Joe's organic shells and white cheddar, brown rice penne pasta, whole wheat pasta
Whole Foods organic pasta varieties, pasta sauce, Neapolitan, Boscaiola

Refrigerated pastas

Buitoni mini-three cheese ravioli, mozzarella and herb tortellini, herb and chicken tortellini
Trader Giotto's cheese tortellini

Pasta sauces

Alessi all-natural marinara pasta sauce
Barilla tomato and basil sauce
Davinci Organics tomato sauce
Enrico's all-natural recipe pasta sauce
Mom's spaghetti sauce
Muir Glen organic tomato pasta sauce
Walnut Acres organic tomato and basil pasta sauce
Whole Kids organic macaroni and cheese, pasta sauce

Rice and dried mixes section

Barbara's mashed potatoes
Fantastic falafel
Lundberg Family Farms organic brown rice
Success brown rice
Texmati 100 percent organic brown rice, brown basmati rice Tilda Brown basmati rice
Trader Joe's organic brown jasmine rice
Uncle Ben's brown rice

Baking section

Arrowhead Mills raw wheat germ, pancake mix
Bob's Red Mill textured vegetable protein, cornmeal
Hodgson Mill organic flours, corn grits/polenta
Krusteaz low-fat oat bran pancake mix

Canned food section

Soups

Amy's organic minestrone soup
Health Valley organic no-salt-added soups, no-salt-added canned tomato varieties
Healthy Choice garden vegetable, country vegetable soups
Imagine organic broths
Pacific organic broths
Trader Joe's organic vegetable broth, chicken broth
Wolfgang Puck's organic hearty vegetable soup

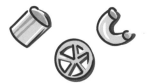

Appendices

Beans
Allens refried beans
Bearitos organic, low-fat, no-salt-
added refried beans, traditional
refried beans
Bush's Best fat-free refried beans
Eden's organic garbanzo beans, pinto
beans, soybeans, refried beans
Rosarita low-fat black bean refried
beans
S&W garbanzo beans, 50 percent
less sodium
ShariAnn's organic refried beans
Trader Joe's organic garbanzo beans,
pinto beans
Walnut Acres organic refried beans
Whole Foods 365 pinto beans,
garbanzo beans

Fish
Bumblebee Wild Alaska pink salmon
Crown Prince pink salmon, low-salt
Denning's red sockeye canned salmon
Trader Joe's organic Wild Alaska pink
salmon

Fruits
Healthy Harvest unsweetened fruit
medleys
Mott's Organics unsweetened
applesauce, no-sugar-added
natural applesauce
Santa Cruz organic unsweetened
applesauce
Trader Joe's organic unsweetened
applesauce
Treetop natural no-sugar-added
applesauce
Whole Kids organic unsweetened
applesauce

Condiments section

Oils and butters
Canola oil brands 100% expeller
pressed
Challenge light butter with canola oil
Land O' Lakes light butter with
canola oil
Nonstick oil sprays (canola, olive,
soy); check sprays for cooking
temperature guidelines
Olive oil brands extra virgin first cold
pressed

Ketchups and soy sauces
Annie's Naturals ketchup
Heinz organic ketchup
Kikkoman naturally brewed lite
soy sauce
Muir Glen ketchup
San-J naturally brewed tamari
Trader Joe's organic ketchup
Westbrae natural ketchup
Woodstock Farms organic ketchup

Syrups and molasses
Grandma's molasses—robust
Maple Grove Farms pure maple syrup
Plantation blackstrap molasses
Springtree pure maple syrup
Trader Joe's organic maple syrup
grade B
Whole Foods 365 Organic 100 percent
pure organic maple syrup grade B

Fruit spreads and nut butters
All Natural Tap'n Apple apple butter
Dickinson's Purely Fruit 100 percent
fruit spread
Knott's Berry Farm 100 percent fruit
spread
Laura Scudders all-natural smooth
peanut butter
Margies 100 percent fruit spread
Sorrell Ridge 100 percent fruit, no
sugar added
St. Dalfour all-natural 100 percent
fruit spread
Trader Joe's organic nut butters and
fruit spreads
Whole Foods 365 fruit spread varieties

Whole Foods 365 Organic smooth almond butter, smooth peanut butter, sesame tahini

Hummus

Cedarlane hummus
Trader Joe's organic hummus dip, tomato basil hummus

Dried fruits section

Regional brands of certified organic raisins, apricots, or mixed dried fruits
Trader Joe's organic Thompson raisins, Blenheim variety unsulphured apricots
Whole Kids organic raisins

Snack section

Ak-Mak 100 percent whole wheat stone ground sesame crackers
Annie's Homegrown baked snack crackers
Barbara's Bakery Wheatines, Raspberry Fig Bars, Organic GoGo Grahams
Calbee Snapea crisps
GenSoy soy crisps (apple cinnamon crunch, rich cheddar cheese)
Hain Pure Foods Wheatettes, carrot chips, popped corn mini-cakes—plain and white cheddar, Mini Munchies
Haute Cuisine organic crackers (varieties)
Health Valley crackers (varieties)
Kashi crackers (varieties)
Koyo organic rice cakes
Lundberg Family Farms organic rice cakes
Manischewitz whole wheat matzos
Mi-Del vanilla snaps
Natural GH Foods Cheddar Guppies
Nejaime's Laasch sesame crisp wafer breads

Our Family Farm Field Friends baked wheat crackers, Captain's Catch baked cheese crackers
Pepperidge Farm crackers (varieties)
Pepperidge Farm Goldfish baked snack crackers (original and 30 percent less sodium cheddar cheese)
Quaker salt-free rice cakes
Roberts American Gourmet Veggie Booty, Pirate's Booty with aged white cheddar
Terra sweet potato chips (no salt added)
Trader Joe's Original savory thins, sesame thins, corn tortilla flat breads, cheese sticks, rich golden rounds, low-fat white cheddar corn crisps, skinny soy chips, soy crisps white cheddar, veggie corn puffs
Tumaro's organic Krispy Crunchy Puffs
Wasa cracker varieties
Whole Foods 365 golden stoneground Wheat Thins—lower-sodium vegetable crackers

Meat section

Bistro Basics

Choose lean ground turkey, turkey breasts, chicken breasts, freshly sliced deli meats.

Aaron's Best ground turkey—Glatt kosher turkey, free-range organic chicken
Applegate Farms organic turkey bacon, organic chicken hot dogs
Diestel Turkey Ranch turkey franks
Foster Farms oven-roasted turkey breast slices
Hans all-natural chicken apple sausage, chicken breakfast links

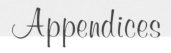

Healthy Choice deluxe think-sliced
oven-roasted turkey breast
Ranger Chicken brand varieties
Trader Joe's natural beef—9 percent fat
ground beef, all natural chicken,
organic free-range chicken,
ground turkey
Wellshire Farms organic turkey bacon

Meat alternatives

(also see Frozen Foods)
Lightlife Smart Franks, Gimme Lean
Sausage Style
Soy Deli organic baked tofu
(honey sesame)
Tofurky oven-roasted deli slices
Wildwood organic baked Aloha tofu
Yves Tofu Dogs, Original Veggie Dogs,
Veggie Sausage Patties, The Good
Deli Veggie Turkey, The Good
Ground Veggie Original

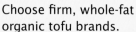

Bistro Basics

Choose firm, whole-fat
organic tofu brands.

Wheat allergy alert! Many
meat substitutes contain
gluten, the allergen in wheat.

Fish section

See First Course, Fishy Fish,
page 29, for good selections,
and the Canned Food section
of this appendix.

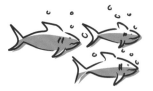

Egg section

Gold Circle Farms DHA omega-3 eggs
Horizon organic eggs
Naturally Preferred organic eggs
Organic Valley omega-3 eggs
Trader Joe's organic grade A free-range
eggs plus omega-3

Cheese section

Bistro Basics

Cheddars containing annatto,
a natural coloring, are fine.

Alpine Lace Jack, provolone,
mozzarella
Alta Dena Organics cottage cheese
BelGioioso sliced mild provolone,
fresh mozzarella
Borden Double Twist
Cabot Vermont white cheddar
Cracker Barrel 2 percent milk
Dubliner Irish cheese
Frigo Cheese Heads Swirls, 100
percent natural string cheese
Horizon organic varieties
Kraft Philadelphia Original or light
cream cheese, Deli Deluxe
part-skim mozzarella, Deluxe
provolone, Twist-Ums
Land O' Lakes mozzarella
Organic Valley varieties
Precious ricotta, string, and
mozzarella cheeses
Sargento varieties
Smart Beat American slices
Sorrento Stringsters
Tillamook Monterey Jack,
cheddar slices

Trader Joe's organic Monterey Jack, organic Vermont white cheddar, Caprese Log, organic mild white cheddar, organic sliced cheddar, yogurt cream cheese, whipped cream cheese, Monterey Jack cheese snack sticks, traditional fresh ricotta, low-fat cottage cheese
Whole Kids string cheese

Cheese alternatives

Bistro Basics

Milk allergy alert! Many cheese substitutes contain casein, the allergen in milk.

Follow Your Heart vegan gourmet cheese
Galaxy Foods veggie slices
Lisanatti Soy-Sation mozzarella style
Soy Kaas mozzarella style, Monterey Jack style
Soyco vegan singles
Tofu Rella cheese and slices
Trader Joe's yogurt cheese, soy cheese mozzarella flavor
Yves Good Slice

Dairy section

Milk
Buy only pasteurized, organic brands of milk. Nonpasteurized milk is a health risk.

Nondairy milks
Eden Soy Extra organic soymilk (shelf stable)

Naturally Preferred organic soymilk
Pacific Ultra Soy plain milk
Organic Valley soymilk (refrigerated)
Silk Soymilk—organic, unsweetened, enhanced
Soy Dream enriched soymilk
Trader Joe's organic soymilk
VitaSoy Complete Original

Yogurt
Dairy yogurts
FAGE Total Greek Style
Helios organic kefir (milk cultured with healthy bacteria and FOS)
Horizon organic yogurt, smoothies
Lifeway kefir, plain
Nancy's organic plain
Oikos organic
Stonyfield Farm organic Yobaby yogurt
Strauss organic plain
Trader Joe's organic yogurt plain, Greek-style plain

Bistro Basics

Look for organic, plain yogurts and sweeten at home with fresh fruit or 100 percent fruit preserves.

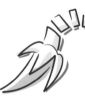

Nondairy yogurts
Nancy's organic soy yogurt (plain)
Silk soy yogurts
Stonyfield Farm O'Soy (all-natural)
Trader Joe's cultured soy plain yogurt
Wildwood Organics soy yogurt (plain)
Wholesoy

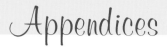

Frozen foods section

Alexia organic oven fries

Amy's organic burgers, organic spinach pizza snacks, organic cheese ravioli, veggie loaf, macaroni and cheese, stuffed pasta shells

Applegate Farms chicken and apple breakfast sausage

Boca organic breakfast patties, links, sausages, burgers

C&W no-salt-added peas, spinach

Cascadian Farms organic frozen fruit or vegetables

Diestel Turkey Ranch pure range ground turkey burgers

Dr. Praeger's fish sticks, spinach pancakes, burgers

Health Wealth chicken patties

Heidi's Hens organic turkey burgers

Lifestream Mesa Sunrise, Soy Plus, 8 Grain Sesame, Flax Plus Toaster Waffles

Morningstar Farms sausage patties, veggie burgers, Chik'n Nuggets, veggie breakfast sausage links

Mrs. Paul's Healthy Selects fish sticks

Naturally Preferred organic mixed vegetables, green beans

Omega Foods salmon burgers

Papa Cristo's spanakopites

Pegasus spinach puffs

Rosina Celentano broccoli-stuffed shells

Seapoint Farms organic edamame

Shelton's free-range turkey sausage patties, meatballs, turkey breast

Sno Pac organic frozen vegetables

Trader Joe's rolled chicken tacos, butternut squash ravioli, chicken pierogi, broccoli and cheddar quiche (remove crust to avoid trans fats), falafels, breaded chickenless nuggets, vegetarian spinach and tofu egg rolls, vegetable samosas, Pilgrim's Pride chicken breast strips (breaded), breakfast patties, low-fat French toast, organic blueberry waffles, frozen organic vegetables, edamame, fruits

Vans organic original waffles, blueberry waffles, 7-grain Belgian waffles, all-natural gourmet multigrain waffles

Vicolo all-natural cornmeal crust pizza

Whole Foods 365 organic cheese lasagna, veggie burgers, vegan burgers, fruit and vegetable varieties

Whole Kids organic mini-waffles, old-fashioned waffles

Whole Ranch lightly breaded fish sticks, fish nuggets

Woodstock Farms organic frozen fruit or vegetables

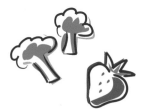

Appendix 3
A blend of measurements

Liquid ingredients

1 cup = ½ pint = 8 fl oz = 236.6 mL
2 cups = 1 pint = 16 fl oz = 473 mL
4 cups = 1 quart = 32 fl oz = 946 mL
2 pints = 1 quart = 32 fl oz = 946 mL
4 quarts = 1 gallon = 128 fl oz = 3.785 L

Dry ingredients

3 teaspoons = 1 tablespoon = ½ oz = 14.2g
12 teaspoons = ¾ cup = 6 oz = 170g
2 tablespoons = ⅛ cup = 1 oz = 28.35g
4 tablespoons = ¼ cup = 2 oz = 56.7g
5 ⅓ tablespoons = ⅓ cup = 2 ¾ oz = 75.6g
8 tablespoons = ½ cup = 4 oz = 113.4g
16 tablespoons = 1 cup = 8 oz = ½ lb = 226.8g
32 tablespoons = 2 cups = 16 oz = 1 lb = 453.6g
64 tablespoons = 4 cups = 32 oz = 2 lbs = 907g

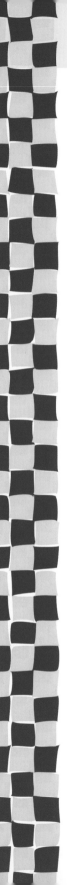

Subject index

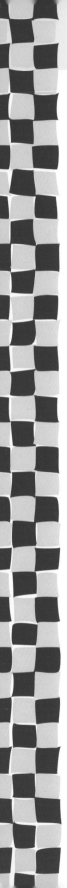

Subject index

Subject index

Recipe index

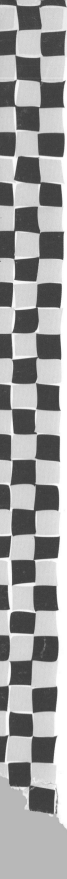

Recipe index